Easy Home Exercises for Seniors Over 60

55 Simple Steps to Stay Strong, Mobile, and Independent

Ross Taosaka

Table of Contents

Introduction

Are we at the beginning of the end?

For many seniors, like you and me, it often seems that as our hair begins to gray and our skin loses its elasticity, or when we retire from our jobs and find it harder to get up from the couch, we give in to thinking that our active lives are nearing an end.

We then find ourselves less inclined to engage in activities that require even modest physical exertion, such as cooking meals and going on hikes. We are older, we tell ourselves, so we simply cannot do as much as we used to. While not being able to leap up a flight of stairs or pop open the pickle jar is perfectly normal as we age, we often forget that we can continue to be active if we do it intelligently and keep ourselves fit.

Aging and its changes do not indicate the end of your life. It merely reveals a new and glorious phase in your years—a new beginning you have rightfully earned.

Then again, that is easier said than done, is it not? We are a species built up of muscles, bones, and the reality of aches and limitations that come with age. We fear the loss of our mobility and independence. We love handling things ourselves. Having to give up that control and having to rely on others and interfere with their own lives, can be depressing and unwanted thoughts. You do not want this to be your reality—not at all.

Instead of addressing these worries directly, we often take the "easy" route of ignoring them without regard to the negative consequences that may result. Others surrender to their decreased strength and mobility, ultimately giving up on moving, exercising, and improving their health. Then some just have no idea where to turn, where to go, or how to get around doing the things they want without getting injured! Perhaps you recognize your current way of thinking as falling into one of these categories. Whatever your reasons and struggles are presented, however, know that with the exercises in this book, you are about to take a different path toward an improved version of yourself.

While there is no fountain of youth to chase and nothing to keep us young forever, there is no reason we cannot remain youthful and active.

The *55 simple steps and exercises* described in this book will provide you with a basic, solid understanding of your body that will silence your fears and allow you to stay strong, mobile, and independent for years to come. With that said, you may be wondering: *Is exercise good for someone like me, too*? Read on, and you'll soon be nodding your head *Yes!* to that question.

What This Book Can Do for You

It is not unusual for people to think that exercise entails complicated and strenuous movements that are dangerous and difficult—especially since we are older. With this book, you will find that exercising, even minimally, will improve your condition and can be a delightful thing to enjoy at any age, even if you have never exercised before.

With clean, straightforward instructions and illustrations, this book will guide you every step of the way on your new journey. Through your efforts, dedication, and realization of your continued vitality, this book will show you how much you can thrive physically, mentally, and emotionally.

Compiled with care, these exercises will allow you to increase strength, gain freedom of movement, lessen pain, and advance yourself in flexibility, balance, and the ability to carry out your daily tasks. By adhering to these exercises and committing yourself to remain strong and mobile, you will find that your everyday tasks and activities, such as showering, dressing, shopping, and traveling, will all become easier than ever!

In summary, my hope is that this book will help you gain renewed impetus to continue engaging in the world around you. My goal in putting this book together is to offer you a brighter outlook on what you, at whatever age you happen to be, can accomplish with more control, freedom, and well-deserved happiness. Live the golden life that you choose for yourself, and let this book be your partner in achieving that.

Using the Book

In writing this book, a number of resources were consulted, such as medical reports, university studies, and exercise journals. This book, therefore, is filled with information and exercises that will help you cope with the changes, declines, and pains we often have to deal with as we age. Treat this book as your guide and companion that will help you get on the road to achieving your goals.

Keep in mind that exercising is not meant to be a contest. There are no "required" criteria to meet or judgments on how fast you must complete the exercises in order to see results. None of that is relevant here. This book is personal to you, to help guide you on your own schedule and at your own pace. Thus, feel no pressure or expectations as you embark on your exercise plan, and I assure you that consistent efforts will give you noticeable benefits.

This book is your personal guide to helping you (and those you share it with) benefit from a healthier life. Anyone, at any level, can reap those benefits. So, take things at your own pace, experience progression over time, and never feel the need to hurry or force anything. Remember to enjoy the process and focus only on yourself. For a moment, allow the world around you to fall silent and fade away. You deserve to look after yourself and live your days significantly, intensely, and without worries, concerns, regrets, or restraints.

From the very moment you searched for a solution and read the first sentence of this book, you were on the right road to caring for and cherishing the only body you have. You took a tremendous step forward in helping your body and mind and to assure a life of being a strong and proud senior—as you should! Follow the book, its steps, and your own heart, mind, and body, and you will know exactly what you have to do.

Author's Authority

In the world we live in now, with so much information (and misinformation) flying around in a frenzied fashion, it is difficult to know what we can truly rely on. You are reading this book now, but you may be wondering whether you can safely place your trust in what I say. This is a very fair concern, indeed. To allay any such fears, allow me to share a bit of my background.

Having been born and raised in Hawaii, I have spent much of my life outdoors, climbing trees, running amok, and exploring the ocean. To live in a place that beckons you to be active, I have learned the importance of a healthy body and a strong, sharp mind.

Fast forward to my college years, where I eventually obtained a law degree and practiced largely in the area of personal injury. This helped me to further understand how injuries happen, the impact that aging has on the body, how our physical selves can heal, and the importance of doing all we can to care for our most important asset—our own bodies.

Later, even while practicing law, I explored other ways to not only understand but to actually take affirmative steps to help and heal injured bodies. As a result, I obtained my license as a Massage Therapist. Being a therapist was and continues to be, an excellent way for me to continue my self-education in physical and mental healing. It reminds me that every person has the same set of muscles and bones but that some of us experience more pain and become less able to move.

Consequently, such limitations can easily lead to a life of having to depend on others and make us hesitant to continue as "fully engaged" members of society. I see this often in people who are injured in accidents or simply because they are older. Even with my 94-year-old mother, I cannot help but sometimes wonder if she would be more mobile if she had engaged in an exercise routine on a daily basis. But please do not worry about mom; she is still the most strong, inspiring, and influential figure in my life!

With hundreds of personal injury and massage clients under my belt, as well as training and experience with Reiki (healing touch) and Aikido (mind and body discipline), I now look at you—yes, YOU—as the next person I want to help.

Selfishly, though, perhaps the one thing that finally spurred me on to write this book is that I care about myself. I, too, am a senior and can absolutely relate to the physical, mental, and emotional changes that occur as we age, ponder our lives, and wonder about what the future holds.

By the way, I do want to point out that caring for yourself is a kind of selfishness that is actually good and highly encouraged. You can do more for others if you are in top-notch condition yourself!

As a Licensed Massage Therapist since 2005, I continue to see people with a wide range of pains, limitations, and, most notably, fears of not being independent in the future. While I certainly cannot guarantee a problem-free existence, I am always encouraged and re-energized each time a client relates how she can now carry her shopping bags without pain or how another client has returned to his favorite activity of paddling outrigger canoes. Nothing is more rewarding to me than seeing such positive results and improvements that allow my clients to thrive.

I treasure helping others heal and better their lives and physical conditions, and I hope to continue doing so for a long time. The role, however, has given me my own challenges to deal with. Massage Therapy itself is very physically demanding. Thus, I need to engage in routine exercises, like the ones discussed in this book, with mental and spiritual drills, too. I am in my 60s, so I know and understand that I need it now, all the more so, and I have to keep a stern eye on my health, as do you.

I am so fortunate to have the opportunity now, after years of experience and training, to share this exercise book with my fellow seniors. I genuinely hope that you will apply what I have written with the brightest and most positive outlook to create for yourself as healthy a life as possible.

Now that I have given you a bit of background on why I have written this book and the experiences that I bring, it is time to turn to you. I hope you are excited and ready to stretch, push, and pull toward physical excellence. Let's get going!

Chapter 1:
Living the Life You Choose

Some may say that growing old means living a life of frailty and weakness and that a loss of strength, mobility, and independence is irreversible and out of our control.

Dear fellow senior, I am here to show you that such thinking can be minimized and overcome. We know that change and consequences come with added birthday candles. The human body transforms, after all, often in ways we do not like, appreciate, or favor. Yet, that does not mean it is all over. Age is just a number when it comes to the ability to improve. You hold the wheel in choosing your lifestyle, hindering the hallmarks of aging, and living the active and fulfilling life you have earned. Through exercise, we can get there together.

How Exercise Helps You Thrive

It is no secret that exercise holds numerous benefits for our health and bodies. Even so, the specific advantages may not always be readily apparent. You might be wondering, "Why should I know this anyway?" and rightfully so. Some of us may not want to sit around reading workout "novels" or medical journals. You came here for the exercises, after all. So I promise to try and keep things brief.

Knowing all the specifics is a way for you to learn and understand more about how your body operates and responds to the work you put in when exercising. This comprehension may also help spark or renew your motivation for the long haul. Knowledge, as they say, is power, and power often leads to action. Action is a necessity when it comes to this journey.

You already have all the potential to brace your feet against the starting blocks; now, you just need the rest of it. Do not worry, though, for I am your starter's pistol: Here to guide and encourage you toward better health. Trust that you have made the right choice in picking up this book, and continue this read with confidence.

Effects on Longevity and Health

What would you say if I were to tell you that exercise slows down aging? Yes, this is a bold claim, but according to recent studies, it seems to be the case. I emphasize the word "seems" because the statement is not only vague but it also encourages people to think positively. No amount of sit-ups or laps will change your chronological age. Then again, nothing can. Your biological age, functional capacity, and quality of life, however, are different stories, and this is where exercise steps in to show its muscle.

It has been well-documented that exercise fights the common effects of aging and optimizes our health in general. In the years to come, it will keep you feeling younger, happier, and healthier while adding to your overall quality of life. When exercise is coupled with other wholesome habits, you hold the key to retaining your energy, vigor, and youthfulness even once you have ripened into a seasoned senior.

Among the many benefits exercises offers, here are a few:

- **Improved immunity**: With age comes increased susceptibility to ailments, infections, and diseases of all sorts as the immune system withers and becomes more fragile. Our bodies are no longer as they used to be; thus, they need all the help they can get, which is why exercise is such an essential part of life. It improves your immune system and contributes to your overall health and well-being. An active lifestyle leads to better sleep, improved moods, lower stress levels, and a healthier, more robust immune system that can help us prevent and manage certain illnesses and conditions, from the common cold to those touching the heart, respiratory system, hypertension, and even certain cancers.

- **Reduces the risk of falls**: Exercise is a great way to prevent and reduce falls by building healthy bones and muscles. This, in turn, improves your overall strength, flexibility, balance, coordination, and posture. Improving on all these aspects helps lessen the likelihood of falls in seniors and non-seniors, even when they may sometimes be unavoidable. You will be active for longer with increased mobility, which will help you sustain the independence and health you treasure.

- **Improves essential parts of the body**: Exercise affects almost every part of our bodies, even down to the cellular level. Our muscles, bones, joints, tendons, and soft tissues, for example, are among those that are influenced and also stand to benefit. All of these form part of our musculoskeletal system, which helps keep our bodies up, moving, and able to do everyday activities. Even our organs benefit from physical activity. In summary, exercise is a great way to ensure that your body and health are in excellent condition, which will help you stay that way, age with grace, and hold onto your mobility and independence as the years come along.

- **Improved sleep and energy**: Getting in plenty of quality, deep, and undisturbed sleep is vital for a healthy lifestyle. Unfortunately, sleep disorders like insomnia, disrupted sleep patterns, and mental health conditions can make it harder for some to obtain this grade of shuteye. One solution that is free and readily available is exercise! While you are active, your body temperature rises, and afterward, it cools down. These changes in your core temperature, along with other contributing factors such as stress reduction and energy utilization, allow you to fall asleep more effortlessly, remain asleep throughout the night, and wake up feeling energized and refreshed.

- **Improved mental health and cognitive function**: You will notice in these exercises that I encourage you to engage your brain and focus on the body part or muscle that is being worked on, to really feel the contraction or stretch that is involved, and to concentrate on making your movements gradual, intentional, and full. Staying physically active and engaging your brain are great ways to improve and benefit your mind and mental health. This may prevent or slow the progression of certain brain and mental health disorders and conditions, such as depression and dementia. Furthermore, as your brain's health increases, your ability to think, learn, react, make decisions, and solve problems is enhanced. Staying mentally sound as you age will be a reality within your reach.

- **Healthier cardiovascular system**: When you exercise, your heart is hard at work, striving to push oxygen into the body and to the muscles you are using. By improving muscle oxygen uptake, we lower the heart's demand to pump more blood to these muscles, thereby decreasing strain on the heart. With less stress hormones, more energy, and stronger muscles and tissues, your overall heart health will improve, and diseases and other bad conditions will be lessened or kept under control.

- **Healthier respiratory system**: With your ticker hearty and healthy, circulation throughout the body is improved, which is a benefit in itself. Fresh blood from your heart sends that crucial oxygen to all parts of your body, from your brain to your toes. This enhanced circulation assures, among other things, more robust tissues and muscles, such as those involved in the respiratory system. Those tissues that benefit include hard tissue (bones), which form your skeletal structure and further helps your breathing and respiratory functioning. It can also help prevent bacteria from entering the respiratory system, ensuring that you can still smell the flowers, breathe deeply without worry, and keep your lungs healthy.

- **Improves endurance**: As mentioned, exercise is a fantastic way to improve and maintain your overall strength, vitality, mobility, and independence as the years add on. Having all these elements and parts in place ensures that you can carry out everyday activities without difficulty, such as interacting with others, playing with your grandchildren, or simply fetching a plate from a higher cupboard. We all want to hold onto our independence and ways of life; with exercise and a healthy life, you can ensure that you hold onto and have exactly that.

Hormonal Benefits

There are four main types of chemicals in your body (hormones) that induce feelings of happiness. Believe it or not, there are ways that exercising and otherwise living with a positive mindset can release these hormones to elevate your mood and make you feel great—especially in times of stress and everyday pressures, for example:

- Dopamine, which is related to reward and motivation, is released when you set goals and reach them. With this book, therefore, set short and long-term goals, and you will be sure to keep your dopamine flowing.

- Serotonin not only assists with digestion, bone health, and sleep but also affects your mood. A great way to increase serotonin is to build your confidence. With exercise, you'll feel better each time you workout and notice that you can do more and more with greater ease as you progress. Confidence leads to more serotonin, which leads to a better mood.

- Oxytocin, endearingly called the "love" hormone, has to do with how you trust other people and bond with them. In our lives, oxytocin is released into our bodies when we kiss, hug, and have sex. It's the reason we feel happy when we cuddle with our pets or develop strong relationships with those we care for. By feeling better about yourself through exercise, you'll interact more with others and develop stronger trust with them. As you develop this, your closeness and intimacy will welcome increased oxytocin.

- Endorphins are commonly known as the "feel-good" hormone that comes with physical exertion. What's a good way to release endorphins? Exercise! Runners get their "high" when endorphins are released during their routines. Even doing the stretches outlined in this book will do the trick. Another good way to get those endorphins flowing is laughter. Have a great time with others as you get in shape, move your body, and laugh out loud. I promise you'll feel great!

How This Book Helps

It was no accident that you found this book and chose to give it a read in the first place: You wanted to find a way to improve and hold onto your strength, mobility, and independence as the years continued, correct? You wanted to achieve this, and perhaps more: A new, reinvigorated outlook on the life you have earned. You choose the life you want to live, after all, and it's all up to you. Now that you have wisely chosen to better yourself, I am here to guide you toward your goals.

As you will see, this book is designed to explain how to perform each exercise, how it benefits you, and why it is essential for improved health. As you engage in each exercise, take note of how your body feels and imagine how it will help you in your daily life.

The exercises presented here are straightforward, easy to follow, and require no special equipment or gym memberships. Moreover, none of the movements are fancy or extreme because a solid understanding of the basics can accomplish the same thing and provide you with the same spectacular results. Even if you are wheelchair-bound or bedridden, many of these exercises can still be performed. This is an exercise book that almost everyone can enjoy, even if you have spent years without exercise.

I surely cannot guarantee you perfect health, but I can state this with confidence: You will experience dramatic improvements physically, mentally, and emotionally when incorporating exercise into your daily routine and accepting this easy-to-use book as your lifelong partner. Together, my fellow seniors, there is much that we can accomplish!

Chapter 2:
Aligning Your Mind and Body

Exercise should not be something difficult to incorporate into your life or to scratch your head about. With simple steps and clear explanations before you, it will instead be as effortless as learning a different hiking trail or trying a new recipe for dinner. Important to any new physical act and lifestyle change, however, is the thinking that goes on in your brain. By aligning your physical body with your mind, your efforts will yield better results with greater staying power. You will sharpen your focus on what you are doing, maintain your motivation, and avoid injuries, too!

The Right Way to Think

It all starts with the attitude and mindset you bring to the table. As the great writer and philosopher Nikos Kazantzakis stated, "To succeed, we must first believe that we can" (Karthik, 2021). The quote says it all: For you to truly excel in your wellness ambitions and growth, you need to have the optimal mindset, attitude, and will not only hold onto your motivation but form habits that last and usher you closer to a healthier, more fulfilling quality of life.

When engaged in any activity in life, your mind and body should be aligned as *one*. Have you ever noticed people looking in one direction but walking in another? Or perhaps with their faces buried in their phones while driving? Those situations never end well. For our purposes, therefore, when it is time for you to exercise, that should be your only concern. Enter into it with good energy and with every intention to better your body.

Even though these exercises are simple and easy, actually getting around to doing them regularly and staying active may be a bit more challenging for some than others. We are often plagued by negative thoughts and feelings, fear of injury, and uncertainties due to health troubles, physical limitations, and other obstacles and concerns. Because of this, we face a higher risk of frequent sedentary deviations or possibly abandoning our fitness goals altogether. We do not want that. Therefore, we must constantly recalibrate our mindset to perform at its best and achieve success.

A positive attitude and mindset will affect how you exercise, rebound from setbacks, handle challenges, remain motivated, attain goals, and maintain general health and wellness. Viewing exercise as "yet another chore" or a simple, tedious activity will not do you any good. With that approach, you will likely not want to do these exercises in the long run because your motivation will run out, and your health will bear the consequences.

Therefore, the first quick tip I have for you today is this: To find triumph in fitness, discover how to genuinely enjoy your workout sessions. Find a way to make them your own, keep a smile throughout, and take it on as an uplifting part of your day simply because it is! With this attitude, and with your mind and body aligned as one, you are already well on your way to bettering yourself.

Not a Fan of Exercise?

Having exercise in my life and seeing the benefits it can provide for my body and health is something I value deeply. In short, I love it! Still, I am quite aware that not everyone shares my perspective and passion.

Whether your dislike of exercise stems from erroneous information, flashbacks of gym class, memories of sore muscles, or plain apathy, many of us choose to avoid physical exertion. It seems so much easier to do nothing, right? Do not feel bad for holding this view, as you are not alone.

From here, we must simply find a way to overcome the notion that exercise cannot be fun, enjoyable, or revitalizing. We can do so by making workouts our own and allowing our physical prowess to shine through in our lives, personalities, and activities.

Whether you decide to do the exercises in this book or take part in any other kind of exercise, here are some suggestions:

- While you exercise, fill your workout space with music that you love, whether it is classical violins or rowdy rock-and-roll. It is *your* space, *your* time, and *your* choice.

- Take your exercise outdoors and do your routine in the sunshine, under a tree, or on your deck. As long as your area is flat, stable, and safe, only your imagination can limit where you exercise. Or, if you are outside, a simple walk and communing with nature can do wonders for your mind, body, and spirit.

- If you happen to be stressed, bored, or just have some time on your hands, try engaging in any physical movement, such as a walk, a nice stretch, or any exercise in this book. Doing so can often be a terrific way to hit the "reset" button and align your mind and body once again.

- Get your friends as excited as you are about exercise, perhaps even inviting them to work through a session together with you. It may evolve into a wonderful way to connect with them on a regular basis. If none of your family members or friends are interested, expand your scope, and meet new people at fitness centers, exercise classes, or other community groups.

- Stay active by spending time with the ones you love; play with your grandchildren, throw a ball for the dog, or meet up with some friends at the local swimming pool.

- Once you learn the various exercises and master them sufficiently, feel free to do them even if it's not time for your normal workout session. Stretch while watching television or videos online, do an exercise while waiting for the kettle to boil, and perform a strength move while talking on the phone. Exercise does not only have to be something you schedule time for. You can incorporate it into many of your everyday activities.

Once you find your positive attitude and are able to bring motivation and energy to your exercise sessions, keep it at the forefront of your mind and ingrain it as your mantra. Be unafraid to try new activities and ways to break a sweat, as you never know what you might like and come to favor. You will soon understand the great satisfaction and even euphoria that exercise can bring, and you will no longer ask, "What if exercise just isn't my thing?"

Preparing Intelligently

Before starting off with your fitness regimen, it would be smart to consider some ways in which you can get started safely while also taking care of and prioritizing yourself throughout.

Involve Your Physician

Although the exercises throughout the book are safe for most people, the adage "better safe than sorry" would apply here where it concerns your precious health. Therefore, if you have any preexisting conditions or health concerns, it might be better to consult a medical professional beforehand. Your healthcare provider can assess your fitness levels, proneness to injuries, general health, and whether certain activities are unsafe for you to perform. It may be a good idea to bring this book along to your next medical appointment to help explain what you intend to engage in. The medical advice you receive will then be more focused and appropriate.

You know yourself best, including what feels right and what may be amiss, whether you are sedentary or active. Paying attention to your body and its changes is vital. While not an exhaustive list, here are some symptoms and conditions that you should heed and perhaps get some medical advice on as you prepare to welcome exercise into your routine:

- Dizziness, lightheadedness, or any difficulty balancing

- Shortness of breath

- Chest pain or pressure in the chest

- Signs of an infection

- Sores that will not heal

- Swollen, red, or tender joints

- Breaking out in cold sweats

- Pain while exercising

- Signs that indicate possible blood clots or other vascular issues

Embracing Exercise

Motivation is an essential part of starting and maintaining your fitness journey. Some of us, however, do find it easier to be self-motivated and committed than others. For those who require a more substantial guiding hand, overcoming this obstacle lies in understanding and recognizing why exercise is good and how it benefits us and those we interact with.

Having already discussed much of that, in the following pages, you will learn even more about the positive impact exercise can have on your life and why it is key to improving your overall quality of being.

You have already taken a critical step by picking up this book with the notion of bettering your body, mind, and spirit. Now that you are on the right road to embracing exercise, you can take the subsequent steps toward making it a part of your routine. Like brushing your teeth, wearing sunscreen, and eating well, know that you are making intelligent choices to move in the right direction. Appreciate your steps, willingness to improve, and courageousness.

I am confident that you will feel the difference once you start these exercises and maintain a regular routine. With each improvement, however slight, you will learn to genuinely enjoy your sessions and look forward to continually building on your accomplishments. As your body responds to your efforts, you will find yourself walking taller with better posture and getting up from the sofa more easily.

With your newfound energy and outlook, other aspects of your life will change, too. You may find it more pleasing to take the longer path while on your walk through the park or that you have more energy to finally clear out that messy closet. Life will be less daunting, and the inevitable obstacles that come your way will no longer seem so overwhelming.

Our main goal should be to view exercise as a well-intentioned, regularly undertaken activity.

You should not see it as something you just "have to do" or take on without giving it much thought. Fully embrace exercise and stay active up to the point where you look forward to every workout and chance of engaging in some kind of healthy movement. Purposefully choose to make it a routine part of your life. So, what are some simple steps to fully embrace exercise?

Here are a few ideas to get you started:

- **Train your brain**: We know that mindset is everything and that with the proper perspective, you can accomplish almost anything. Changing your mindset to recognize and acknowledge that you deserve a better, healthier lifestyle is, therefore, essential for genuinely embracing your exercise routine. Focus on areas of your life that make you feel good, like eating more greens, meditating, or spending more time with family and friends. Find something healthy and enjoyable. Be innovative and do what makes you happy.

- **Understand the true meaning of a *good workout***: Exercise is often confused with something that has to leave every muscle achingly sore, exhausted, and drained for days. It should not be like that at all. Instead, you should feel energized, relaxed, and restored (although the first few sessions might not seem like it at first). Listen to your body and how exercise makes you feel, as you are more likely to adhere to a routine that makes you feel good. Rest whenever you feel the need to and embrace each workout with the thought of how it will make you feel afterward. Look forward to your sessions and ensure that you are moving safely and responsibly.

- **Observe and reflect**: We know that exercise holds various advantages, but without benefits that are significant, undeniably clear, or with a direct focus, we often miss what we are gaining from our workouts. Identifying and noting these physical, mental, and emotional changes you feel and see over time is of great advantage to you. It will help you embrace exercise and want to stay active even more. Do you have more energy and mobility while playing with your grandchildren? Is it easier for you to pick things up and carry them around? Are you more comfortable while exercising? Reflect on all these changes and notice how you are getting healthier.

- **Scheduling**: As any routine implies, it is up to you to find the time to exercise. Commit to and accept exercise as part of your lifestyle by setting up and adopting a schedule that ensures you exercise regularly. It does not mean you have to cut out time, activities, and events that you enjoy doing; just make sure to leave an open slot for working out and try your best to stick to it with regularity.

Comfort Is Key

When engaging in these exercises, you must focus on completing them correctly, thoroughly, and safely. The last thing you want or need are clothes that bind or irritate you. As in sports or any other physical activity, what you wear should help to promote your optimal performance.

Proper exercise attire should prevent injuries, enhance mobility, ensure comfort, prevent skin irritation, increase confidence, and improve overall endurance, power, and recovery. So, whether it be your favorite pair of leggings, a comfy tee, or those freshly-washed sweatpants right out of the dryer, the choice is yours! Just ensure that you choose clothes that allow for freedom of movement, which will put you in your happy place.

Your shoes, and whether you decide to wear any, depend on your exercise area and preferences. If you wear shoes, ensure that they allow for stability and provide good support. Your choice of the shoe should work for you with respect to any mobility or physical issues you may have. You should not experience any pain or discomfort while exercising. If your shoes hurt you or make you feel uncomfortable while exercising, it would be best to change your footwear. Wearing socks without shoes is probably not the best idea, as you will be more likely to slide, slip, and lose your balance. Sometimes, depending on your exercise space, doing your workout in bare feet is the best and most comfortable option!

In addition to feeling free and comfortable in your clothes, you should also be comfortable in the room in which you exercise. To enhance your safety and freedom, maintain a clean, clutter-free space (to prevent trips and falls) without distractions and ensure your personal space is your own for the duration of the workout.

Focus on your goals for each particular day and which exercises you will be doing. Engage in them with an optimistic outlook and a joyful attitude. Remember, embrace exercise!

Say Hi" to Hydration

Water is widely known to be essential for a healthy and well-run body. Therefore, combining hydration with exercise can be seen as a sort of dynamic duo for optimizing our physical and mental functioning.

Here are some of the ways in which good hydration benefits you:

- Allows for the optimal performance of the body.
- Sustains high functioning of your mind, concentration, and mental health.
- Maintains and increases endurance.
- Prevents excessive heart rate elevations.

- Maintains performance and energy levels.

- Reduces heat exhaustion and stress.

- Maintains a healthy heart and blood flow thereby providing strong brain and muscle support.

- Reduces muscle injuries, muscle spasms, and overall soreness.

- Supports muscle movement, overall mobility, and recovery.

- Aids in the removal of body toxins.

According to dietitian Allie Wergin (2022), approximately 60% of the human body is water. Clearly, proper hydration is needed to keep our blood flowing, organs functioning, joints lubricated, temperatures regulated, and oxygen dispersed throughout our entire system.

While we exercise, there is a rise in our body's temperature, which causes us to perspire. This is the body's way of obtaining an optimal temperature by releasing fluid to remove heat. Through this process, you lose water, which is vital for your body and health.

Water loss while exercising can result in serious problems, such as dehydration, muscle fatigue, excessive sweating, heat stroke, and other mental and physical declines. Therefore, replacing these fluids by drinking enough water before, during, and after working out is essential. Keeping a water bottle with you during exercise will be a useful reminder to replenish this loss of water and ensure that your body continues humming along like a well-calibrated machine.

Breathing for Life

Yes, as the heading reminds us, we are, quite literally, alive because we breathe. We breathe non-stop every day, so it is nothing foreign to us. It has been there from the moment we were born, and since then, we have rarely given it much thought. But why would we? Breathing is just a simple inhale and exhale, right? In reality, it is more complex than just that.

People often adopt the wrong techniques and ways of breathing, especially when working out. When exercising, we try to focus on what we are doing right, wrong, and everything in between. We work our muscles and raise our heart rates, and we sweat, sometimes a lot, and it can be a messy deal, which is where our breathing often falls off.

In a gym, for example, you will hear people wheezing and groaning or sometimes stopping breathing from forcing an exercise movement. Obviously, these types of breathing are less than optimal when we are relaxed, but not surprising at all when we exert ourselves. In doing the exercises in this book, you will note that I often remind you to breathe. There are reasons why proper breathing, whether you are exercising or not, is essential to good health. Here are some key points to keep in mind:

- **Weight watching**: Glucose, or blood sugar, is our body's primary source of energy (Dolson, 2006). It can be used either immediately or stored for later, whereafter it is known as glycogen. When the body is not getting glucose from food or when we are stressed, it uses glycogen to release glucose into the bloodstream. Only after glycogen is exhausted will the body start burning fat. This is especially problematic for those struggling with high numbers on the scale and wanting to enhance their health by shedding pounds. When we have a surplus of oxygen, our bodies trigger a "relaxation response" of sorts. This helps us switch from glycogen to stored fat and helps us burn it more efficiently for fuel. This allows us to regulate and lose weight more effortlessly and efficiently. Additionally, breathing increases our cardiovascular capacity, which allows us to enhance the benefits of exercise and burn more fat cells when involved in cardio training.

- **Carbon Detoxification**: Certainly, you have heard about how we take in oxygen and release carbon dioxide. In fact, you are expelling it from your body at this very moment. It is a natural waste gas that, when we breathe, moves from our blood to the lungs before being breathed out. Frequent and consistent removal of it from the body is critical. Incorrect breathing patterns make it harder for our bodies to expel this waste, which weakens our bodies and makes us more susceptible to diseases. Breathing correctly will not only allow effective removal of this waste but will also improve your posture as filling your lungs straightens and lengthens the spine.

- **Optimal Body Chemistry**: When we experience pain, there is much that a breath or two can assist with. Breathing allows us to release endorphins, or chemicals, into the body, which helps cure us of ailments, pains, and aches naturally. As breathing also activates the "relaxation response" and increases neurochemical production in the brain, you will be left feeling calmer and happier in no time. You could almost say that it is a natural drug of sorts.

- **Enhancing energy**: Breathing increases blood flow which cleanses the body of toxins and debris, relieves stress, and improves circulation, sleep quality, and stamina. All of these factors contribute to a greater increase in energy and a more efficient use of that energy.

- **General care**: Breathing deeply is a great way to improve our overall health and wellness by increasing and enhancing various processes and systems within our body. For example, when we breathe properly, we clean the blood, cells, and tissues within the body while removing toxins and waste. This also allows our digestive systems to work more efficiently due to improved circulation and a calmer nervous system. Our lymphatic system, which relies on oxygen to move and work properly, is boosted through the increase of oxygen levels, which better protects us from illnesses, maintains bodily fluids, absorbs fats, and removes cellular wastes.

Clearly, breathing correctly is essential for our health. We need to do so properly to ensure we are truly reaping the benefits from both it and exercise. Thus, inhale and exhale with intent as you work through your movements while remaining comfortable, relaxed, and at ease.

Mind Your Mindfulness

For each of these exercises, whether you find them to be easy or challenging, here are a few things to keep at the forefront of your mind.

Know yourself and your limits. In our effort to continually improve, it is good to raise the bar a bit each time so that you challenge yourself. Do this safely, however, to avoid injury and pain to the remarkable vessel that is your body. As you begin these exercises, stay mindful of your health, limitations, fitness levels, and all the messages your body tries to send you. For example, stop immediately if you experience any pain or discomfort. Your body is clearly trying to tell you something is amiss or that you are pushing yourself too far.

Take things easy and build your strength as you progress through each exercise and over time. Focus only on doing your personal best, regardless of whether you can complete the workout or movements in their entirety. Exercise of any kind is worthwhile and beneficial. All you have to do is be patient, not force anything, and enjoy your sessions. Remember that taking things slow, persevering, and improving each time will provide you with the best results, or as the saying goes, "the slow and steady, wins the race."

Still, aim to complete the exercises as deliberately and thoroughly as you can manage; do not rush through the workout. Take your time and concentrate during your sessions. Observe how your body feels as you move, the pace of your breathing, and the way your muscles expand, contract, and relax.

Ensure that you follow the instructions carefully and refer to the illustrations to identify what you are working on and why the exercise is beneficial. Focus, intention, and purpose should guide every move you make.

Your exercise routine is not simply going through the motions described in this book. It includes the pre-exercise setting of your mind, the actual exercising, and, very importantly, the post-exercise recovery period. If your muscles ache a bit the next day or two, that may actually be a good sign that your body is improving. You are alive, and you are feeling it! If you are in great pain, maybe you pushed yourself too far and would need to take time to rest. In any circumstance, listen to your body and use common sense.

In light of safety concerns, I also wanted to mention the following: These exercises are meant for everyone, and many of them can be done while seated. Therefore, even if you have limited mobility or are wheelchair-bound, you can participate and reap the benefits by using a chair. However, ensure that you choose a robust and sturdy seat with a backrest and no wheels (or locked wheels) when exercising. A chair that will remain strong and stationary will keep you from sliding around and falling in the middle of an exercise.

This is the best way to ensure that you are comfortable, safe, protected, and in the best position to perform these exercises well. Thus, if ever during the workouts you find yourself sitting, know that an appropriate chair is essential. Some exercises call for armrests, while they may get in the way of others. See whether the instructions clue you in on which one you need to use, whether you can use a chair with armrests, and whichever is most comfortable when the choice is up to you. The chair must be reliable and meet the requirements discussed above to ensure you carry out the exercises without injuring yourself or jeopardizing your exercise.

Other options that you can experiment with depending on your needs might include handrails, non-slip mats, or cushions. It is always better to be safe than sorry, and being creative about your physical activity is always encouraged.

A Balanced Lifestyle

From the time we learned to take our first steps to ride bicycles and traverse trails, we knew and understood the meaning of one word—balance. The ability to balance has always been a vital and crucial part of our everyday lives. Without proper balance, we could not function as we do.

Some may have the misconception that certain people are simply prone to having poor balance and that nothing can be done to improve that. We easily jump to assigning labels to ourselves or others, such as clumsy, inattentive, or having two left feet. Fortunately, those viewpoints are erroneous, as there is much we can do mentally and physically (as you will see!) to keep ourselves better balanced.

Taking the concept of physical balance further, there is also much that we can do to balance our lives and lifestyles on a broader scale. Exercise and physical activity are just one part of your interesting and multifaceted life. As you venture forward with your workouts, do not forget to balance them with proper food consumption, mental calmness and clarity, intellectual fulfillment, and a healthy sense of your place in this world.

You Are What You Eat

A healthy body starts with what we consume. Filling your plate with the right foods and nutrients is the foundation for overall health and well-being. Diet plays a significant role in maintaining body weight, sustaining bodily functions, raising energy levels, and boosting mood and memory, among other things. Still, sometimes "eating right" is easier said than done, especially if you have a sweet tooth or a lingering eye for fries. These challenges, however, can be overcome by implementing gradual modifications in your eating choices. This will not only further aid your physical endeavors but also allow you to finally uplift your entire body holistically. Here are some things to think about as you plan your future meals:

- **Knowing your recommended intakes**: Knowing what "healthy eating" looks like can be challenging lately, especially with all the fad diets and eating rumors. The Healthy Eating Plate, fortunately, is an excellent detailed guide that helps people make wiser, more nutritious choices when choosing the right foods. The Healthy Eating Plate was created by Harvard Health Publishing and nutrition experts at the Harvard School of Public Health. It is based on the most up-to-date nutrition research, and it is not influenced by the food industry or agriculture policy (Harvard University, 2019). You can find it at: https://www.health.harvard.edu/staying-healthy/healthy-eating-plate.

- With every food group represented, it assists you in producing healthy, balanced meals packed with variety. Using this plan will require you to consume half of your plate as fruits and vegetables, a quarter as whole grains, another quarter as proteins, and a moderate amount of healthy plant oils. Additionally, keep in mind your own dietary needs, including any restrictions or demands like diabetes, high cholesterol, and lactose intolerance.

- **Learning your limits**: Try cutting back on certain foods or avoiding them altogether as you age, such as those high in saturated fats. Foods high in sodium and caffeine are also not advisable for those with a history of hypertension, anxiety, heart conditions, and problems sleeping. Sugary foods and drinks, such as sodas, can raise blood sugar levels, contributing to various health concerns such as obesity. Also, keep an eye on your medication and the foods that could interfere with them. Grapefruits, for example, can intensify the effects of high blood pressure medications and those treating insomnia and anxiety.

- **Make your calories count**: Our metabolisms decrease as we age. This can be problematic as we often do not change the amounts or types of foods or calories we consume, which is often too high for the metabolism to work through. Despite our efforts to reduce our calorie consumption, our need to obtain necessary nutrients sometimes leaves a surplus of calories the body cannot handle. Working off these additional calories, especially at our age, can be particularly challenging. Coupling the proper diet with your exercise plan is an excellent way to ensure that what you put on your plate counts toward your overall well-being. Also, avoid consuming any "empty" calories that give you no benefits, such as those we get from fast foods. Sticking to the foods in The Healthy Eating Plate's recommendations will make it easier for you to navigate through what you consume.

- **Do the research and know your weaknesses**: Take some time to analyze and identify the weaknesses within your diet. Some of us might not be aware of the number of ruinous foods we consume as we often do not pay attention to our eating habits or know which foods are the right ones for us. Thus, research can help you immensely and even make eating healthy more fun! You could, for example, read up on all the different foods you can buy, recipes you can make, and the various combinations that work with your body and age. Knowledge is key to understanding your body and what it needs to help you along your journey toward better health. So, if you have a soft spot for sugary drinks, slowly swap them out for flavored water or herbal teas, or if you are a fan of dairy, replace them with healthier variations. Changes, whether big or small, will take you a long way.

Silence Stress And Find Your Freedom

Stress is a prominent contributor to decreased health and the development of all sorts of ailments and conditions. Stress and negative feelings keep us from truly enjoying our lives and all they have to offer. Thus, taking the time to address your stressors, improve your outlook on life, and take care of yourself is a must, especially when your health and happiness are at stake. Through the proper management of tense or negative thoughts and feelings, you can enhance your health and maintain the proper way of living happily.

To ensure that you have all of these things under your belt as you age, here are some suggestions you can follow:

- **Make time to de-stress and relax daily**: Whether it is waking up in the morning to savor the sunrise, scheduling time in the afternoon to focus on quiet meditation, or ending your day thinking about what you are grateful for, making a continuous effort to relax and work through your stress is critical. Stress and related problems often accumulate over time, making it hard to identify and specify what is causing you trouble. Therefore, try to stay consistent in your thoughts, emotions, and stress management efforts. As previously stated, where your mind and body should be one, de-stressing your mind will do the same for your body.

- **Indulge in your outlets**: Make time to do things you love and find ways to coddle yourself with activities and things that help you relax. You could try something new or lay focus on your hobbies, such as listening to music, reading, writing, or simply spending time outdoors. Get creative, take classes, learn new skills, and try new things when you can to really focus on your health and improve it while you're having fun.

- **Make everyday activities more fun**: When you do the same thing day after day, it can become tedious and unrewarding, especially when you are stressed. Therefore, try to make every task and chore you have as enjoyable as possible. Try out new recipes, take long aromatherapy baths, stroll through the park, and wash your dishes with more gusto. This might take more creative thought, but I am sure you will find your way.

- **Release and reset**: It can be helpful to let out all of your thoughts and emotions so that you can let go of what you are carrying around and what is causing you stress. You can keep a journal where you write down your emotions and thoughts as you experience them and as they come up. Or, try keeping a digital log, video diary, or share your thoughts with a good friend or professional. You know what would be most suitable for you and would act as the best way for you to express what you are experiencing and feeling. Sharing your thoughts and feelings may soon find you feeling less stressed and better able to cope with whatever life throws your way.

- **Pursue professional aid**: You might consider seeking therapy or counseling if some stressors or feelings inhibit your ability to function as well as you'd like. A professional, trained to guide people who occasionally need a stable and experienced hand, can help you work through your challenges and manage your stressors effectively—now and for the long term. Mental therapy for your mind is just as effective as physical therapy for your body.

- **Cut out your stress**: Many things in life add to and aggravate our stress levels. Sometimes, removing these stressors altogether is the best approach. Whether you want to spend more time away from the digital world, stop drinking alcohol, or change some habits, this is all up to you. If you feel that removing things from your life is the best way to achieve happiness, go for it! Remember, you live the life that you choose.

- **Prioritize staying active**: A healthy lifestyle where stress is effectively managed starts with physical activity. Do the exercises discussed in this book as regularly as possible and attempt to stay consistently active. Your body takes a significant hit when you are stressed. When you work on your physical health and eat properly, you release tension from your frame while allowing your body to recover and regain its ability to receive a heightened sense of wellness and joy.

Stay Social

I sometimes run across articles and blogs advancing the idea that seniors prefer cutting their ties, living alone, and socializing as little as possible. The way I see it, however, this is not the truth! We are a social species designed with the desire for connections and relationships, whether we make friends or spend time with family members. Age does not change this. Socializing and maintaining relationships are integral in ensuring you live a balanced life where you are mentally and even physically healthy. Having these healthy relationships in your life allows you to feel happy and content as your sense of worth and belonging increases while symptoms of depression, anxiety, stress, and loneliness decrease.

Here are a few quick ideas on how you can make your connections last:

- Take the initiative by contacting your friends and scheduling get-togethers with family members.

- Take a class or workshop to learn new skills or information and meet those trying to do the same. You could even start a class or social group to share workouts using this very book!

- Volunteer at shelters, charities, and events that match your interests and abilities. It is a great way to feel more fulfilled and make a difference while meeting people with similar goals and objectives.

- Browse online for support groups, chat rooms, and social media platforms. You never know who you'll meet or what connections you'll make all over the world.

- Reconnect with people from your past. Find out what their life is like, what they have been up to, or how their dog is doing. You might spark some old connections and become great friends again, or at least contribute to another person's happiness that you thought of them and reached out.

More Ideas for Better Balancing

The exercises discussed in the book are focused on stretching your muscles and strengthening them. They address and focus on specific muscles and movements. However, you should never limit yourself to doing only one thing. Finding as many ways to stay active as possible is a great way to increase your health and overall quality of life. With that in mind, be bold in finding different avenues toward your goal of incorporating exercise and movement into your life. Once you get used to being more physically active, your mind will also shape itself into being more forward-thinking as well.

Finding new and creative ways to exercise is easy once you open yourself to it. In the meantime, here are some ways to increase your physical mobility, strength and health beyond the exercises in the book:

- **Opt for walks when and where you can**: These days, we tend to travel, run errands, and move around in the comfort of our cars. Why not break out of that passive mode and instead use the opportunity to employ your legs? Walk to the store, take strolls with friends, meditate on an easy hike or bicycle to the park.

- **Put on some music**: Draw the curtains and dance around your home or while doing chores. Even a simple shuffle will do just fine. Dancing is a great form of aerobic exercise that allows you to relieve stress and enjoy yourself. There are also various classes you can take and online videos you can watch for inspiration and guidance. Whatever your ability, dance like nobody's watching!

- **Take your time**: Whether you are out shopping, walking the dog, running an errand, or just enjoying a scenic stroll, immerse yourself in everything around you, proceed at an unhurried pace, and be mindful of the interesting people and activities going on around you. If you are not on a tight schedule, take the time to appreciate and be grateful for all that surrounds you. You will probably notice your heart rate slowing down, a calmer sense of peace, and a brighter view of the world.

- **Choose healthier options**: I know that sometimes we do not want to take the stairs or walk the dog, but choosing these options is much better for your health. Therefore, aim to make healthier choices as often and as regularly as you can, even when your motivation may be lacking. Just like with exercising, you will soon find yourself more easily opting for these better choices. As is often the case, the hardest part is to simply take that first step.

- **Be an opportunist**: When you are sitting up in bed, watching your favorite show, brushing your teeth, or standing at the microwave waiting for your food, you have the perfect opportunity to stay active. Instead of just biding your time, avail yourself of one of the easier exercises (if it is safe to do so) such as doing calf raises while the microwave growls or some of the seated exercises while you are on the couch. If there is an opportunity to exercise, take it!

Build Up Your Exercise Routine

Starting a new exercise routine can be confusing, especially when you have not exercised in years or never even thought about an exercise regimen until today. The only effort you should have to make to begin, however, is to understand why exercising is helpful, and how to do it; the rest should come easily.

Thus, here are some suggestions that will help you construct your exercise routine:

- **Set a specific goal**: Staying true to your exercise motivations can be daunting. Even though you might have your primary goal in sight (your main reason for wanting to change your lifestyle), the journey will not be accomplished overnight. So, where does one begin? By setting smaller goals, you lay down the steps needed to climb to the top of your ladder and toward your main objective. If you started exercising to be more mobile and join a yoga class, for example, first set up reasonably reachable goals such as being easily able to touch your toes within a week or go an hour-long bicycle ride within a month. These goals will help you find direction in your journey, harness motivation when needed, and set yourself up for success.

- **Determine your personal reason for exercising**: Identify the reasons you decided to exercise. Was your family your inspiration? Did health concerns give you a scare? Or are you simply doing it to become a happier, healthier version of yourself? Know your "because" and "why," and it will motivate you in the long run. Remind yourself of these reasons when you feel unmotivated.

- **Resist an all-or-nothing mindset**: Any exercise is good exercise, no matter how small it might seem. Remember to take things at your own pace, progress with time, and do only as much as your body allows.

- **Couple your exercise with something uplifting and motivational**: Spend time in a healing atmosphere with yourself or your workout partners, listen to your favorite music, or simply relish your beautiful surroundings.

- **Have patience**: Solid benefits do not happen overnight; they take time. Just keep pushing forward and continue putting in the work. Sooner or later, the results will follow, and I promise you they will be worth it!

- **Be kind and loving to yourself**: We are often our harshest critics. We tend to be hard on ourselves when things are rough or do not go our way. Overcome this and love yourself at all times. Give yourself compliments in the morning, pat yourself on the back after completing an exercise, and cherish the accomplishments you make along the way. Know that you deserve it!

Keep all of these thoughts, tips, and bits of information in mind as you embark on your exercises. Review them occasionally to remind yourself of your proper mindset, how to make the most of your sessions, and to keep you on track in your physical endeavors and overall life. While this book will serve as a trusted resource, it will also be there as your life-long friend and companion. Confide in it when you feel the need!

Chapter 3:
Why You Should Stretch

Have you ever seen videos of animals in the wild engaging in long, deep stretches? Or perhaps you have seen cats and dogs having a good, relaxing yawn as they elongate their bodies before carrying on with their day. Even kings of the jungle, such as lions, take the time to stretch, relax, and lengthen their muscles. As human beings and members of the animal kingdom, those same reasons apply to us, too. We need stretching in our lives, and here's why.

The Benefits of Stretching

A common problem we face as seniors is the fear of losing our mobility and independence. The U.S. National Institute on Aging reports that seniors lose their independence more from inactivity than from aging itself. From the benefits of exercise alone, we know that staying active is a great way to prevent this loss and improve overall health. So, what are the contributions that stretching brings to the table?

Stretching has long been known for averting injuries and improving muscle flexibility, which is, in itself, hugely beneficial. Increased flexibility makes it easier to move about and live your day-to-day life as you please. However, flexibility and preventing injuries are but two of a number of benefits to be realized. Stretching holds various benefits for the body and allows us to work at our best and remain *autonomous*.

Here are some other ways in which stretching contributes to daily living:

- **Increased range of motion**: For joints to remain healthy, they must move through their full range of motion every day. If not, there will be a resultant insufficiency in the flow and circulation of synovial fluid (a thick, nutrient-rich liquid that lubricates and reduces friction between joints while cushioning the bones). As a result of decreased synovial fluid, we may suffer from stiff, dysfunctional, and degraded joints, with an overall decreased range of motion and mobility. When you stretch, you extend soft issues and allow joints to move through their full range of motion. This allows synovial fluids to circulate and coat the joints, making it easier for you to move and hold onto your mobility.

- **Improved posture**: Poor posture happens gradually, often without us noticing, such as when we spend years slumped in front of desks or hunching over computers. Before we know it, we are slouched over with weak, imbalanced muscles that ache. With stretching and strengthening exercises, you help to work and reinforce these muscles, align the body, regain stability, remove discomforts, and contribute to an even more improved range of motion.

- **Increased circulation**: Poor circulation and blood flow within the body can result in various tribulations such as tingling, numbness, fatigue, pain, or cramps within extremities. It may also manifest itself in cognitive dysfunctions, fluctuations in temperature, pale or blue skin, and a decrease in recovery time. Stretching is a great way to combat these concerns by improving circulation and blood flow throughout the body. Blood vessels open up when you stretch, which allows blood, oxygen, and nutrients to flow more freely and in greater volume to the muscles. If you are fortunate enough to get massages on occasion, those sessions working in conjunction with stretching are an ideal way to move your fluids, distribute oxygen-rich blood, and rid your body of toxins.

- **Prevention and recovery**: The benefits of warming up your muscles before exercise are numerous. By stretching, you ensure that your muscles are loose and ready for any activity by, among other things, increasing flexibility and blood flow. This also means that muscles are more pliable, compliant, and less likely to tear, which is where the idea of "stretching helps prevent injuries" comes from. Stretching, when done right, is a great way to warm up and prepare for your workout; stress and strain are avoided, and muscle tension and soreness are released beforehand. Stretching also ends your workout on a positive note by allowing your muscles to cool down and for you to ease into a relaxed state of mind—that's right, aligning your mind and body! If you stretch after your workout, your heart rate and breathing calm down, your blood flow increases, and your oxygen and nutrient dispersion to your body and muscles is enhanced which later aids in recovery. As a word of caution, although stretching to begin your workout is great, be careful not to overstretch your cold muscles. When we have a lot of energy at the beginning of our workouts, we may tend to push hard and take it too far. Easy does it; just enough to get your blood flowing and muscles primed.

- **Reduced risk of falls**: Stretching, as we know, allows you to adopt a better posture, which also helps you regain stability. This, in other words, means that you will have better balance on your side as you realign your frame and correct imbalances. As your muscles are also working more efficiently, you will be able to enhance your coordination. These improvements, along with other contributors, promote bone health and strength, which allows them to work as they should, if not better.

- **Diseases and prevention**: It is no secret that stretching greatly enriches our general health. In fact, the extent of it is so significant it is said to delay the onset of some conditions and diseases, such as those affecting the vascular system. Some stretches press onto the blood vessels, which releases chemicals that open the arteries and allow blood to enter and flow more freely. This protects us against heart diseases, strokes, diabetes, and other conditions associated with a lack of blood flow. Stretching may also reduce muscle cramps, lower blood pressure, and manage symptoms and pains, such as those associated with arthritis. Furthermore, you might just notice an overall improvement in your quality of life due to an increase in vitality, health, and disease management.

- **Mental enhancements**: The benefits of stretching extend not only to your physical health but also to your mental well-being. Stretching and getting in touch with your body allows you to enter a state of relaxation where you not only unwind but allow yourself to focus more intently and mindfully on your workout. Physically, you are also "unwinding" mental exhaustion from your body. Stress, whether emotional or physical, causes our muscles to tighten. Stretching will help your mind and your body to be free of strain and disorder. It helps relieve pressure and tension from the muscles and body. Furthermore, you might notice an upsurge in energy due to the rise in oxygen, blood, and nutrients within the body, which can aid performance and help you take on your day with more vibrancy.

Clearly, we can all gain a thing or two from stretching. In fact, I have only scratched the surface of the benefits you can reap. When combined with other exercises, such as those you will read about later, you will come to find that your exercise regimen will become an unstoppable force, fit to make your everyday life easier and your health better than ever.

Chapter 4:
Stretching Your Upper Body

Neck Forward Flexion

How This Helps You

Neck sore after you slept? This exercise will help undo that. This exercise helps loosen the strap-like muscles in the posterior or back of the neck that helps you extend and rotate your head. In addition to removing tension, this exercise allows your neck muscles to become more flexible, stress-resistant, limber, and more prone to shaking off any pain. It is the perfect exercise for those who struggle with sore neck muscles or have difficulty shifting their head position because of tightness. Doing this exercise routine will allow greater freedom to perform even simple tasks like looking down to tie your shoelaces.

How to Do It

1. Stand tall or sit up straight. Remaining relaxed, bring your chin down toward your chest as far as you can.

2. Feel the stretch in your cervical spine at the back of your neck and hold it for 5 seconds before returning to your starting position. Repeat for a total of 10 times.

As you advance, place your hand on the back of your head and use it to gently lower your chin down even more. Do not overdo it, bring it down too much, or hurt yourself. Do attempt, however, to feel the natural relaxation of your neck muscles as you hold the stretch for longer.

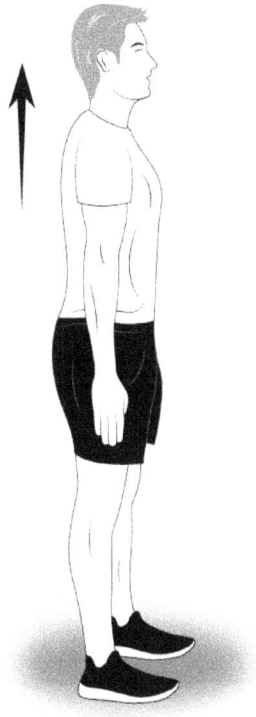

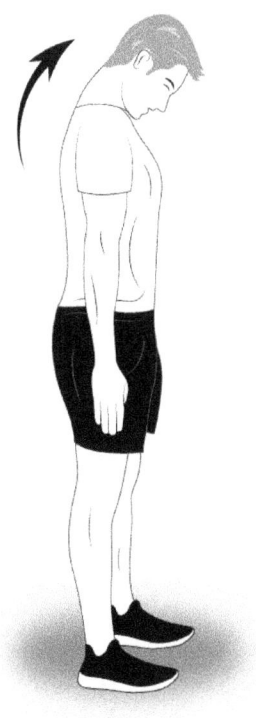

Neck Side Flexion

How This Helps You

As with the Neck Forward Flexion exercise above, Neck Side Flexion exercises help loosen the neck by working on its lateral or side muscles. This will also give you more flexibility and make it easier to move around. It will also make your neck less painful and stiff. As a result, you will have more control when moving your neck and head, with comfort to last.

How to Do It

1. Stand or sit up with your back straight while facing forward. Try obtaining a proper posture while still remaining comfortable.

2. Slowly tilt your head to the right, bringing your right ear down toward your shoulder as far as you comfortably can while only moving your head. Your shoulder should remain still.

3. If you feel comfortable doing so, you may use your hand to guide your neck further down but prioritize your safety and do not force things. Remember that even the smallest of moves can still be effective, and even slightly overdoing it can cause injury.

4. Hold this stretch for 5 seconds. While doing so, narrow your focus onto the feeling of the left side muscles lengthening and loosening as they stretch.

5. Slowly return your head to the starting position before repeating the movement on the left side, stretching the neck muscles on your right.

6. Repeat the stretch a total of 10 times on each side. Take things slowly; do not rush through these movements, and ensure you do them completely and with purpose.

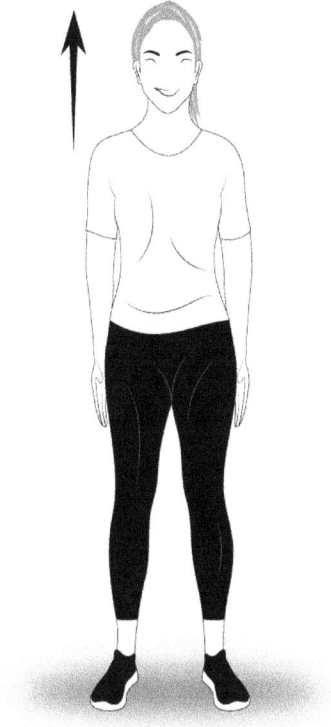

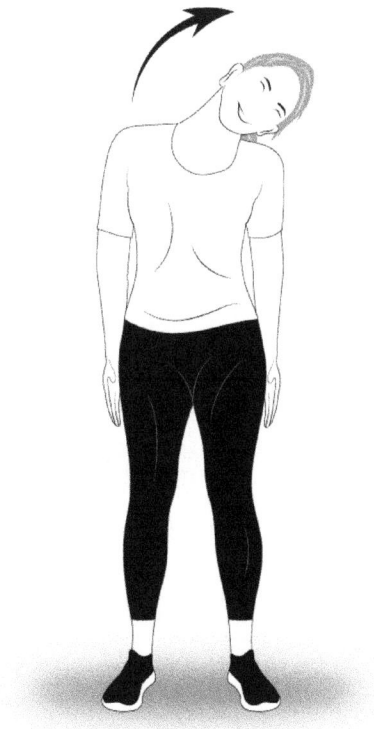

Neck Rotation

How This Helps You

This exercise will help you rotate your neck as it targets and loosens both the back and side muscles of the neck. With this stretch, you should experience greater flexibility and ease of movement in the neck and head. You will also find that some actions, such as pulling out of your driveway or peeking over your shoulder, will become easier and more comfortable over time. We spend the majority of our time looking straight ahead. This often means that we neglect to work our other neck muscles sufficiently. By doing Neck Rotations regularly, you will open the door to a more relaxed way to view the beautiful world around you.

How to Do It

1. Stand tall or sit up straight with your shoulders relaxed while facing forward.

2. Gently turn your head to the right as far as you comfortably can. As you are doing so, try to identify and focus on a single spot as far behind you as possible. Move slowly, take your time, and truly appreciate the feeling of your neck muscles extending.

3. Hold for 5 seconds before returning to the starting position.

4. Repeat on the other side by turning your head to the left and finding a new focal point.

5. Repeat for a total of 10 times on each side. Do not rush through these rotations. Remember that doing a stretch quickly does not make it more effective. Just relax and enjoy the new perspective!

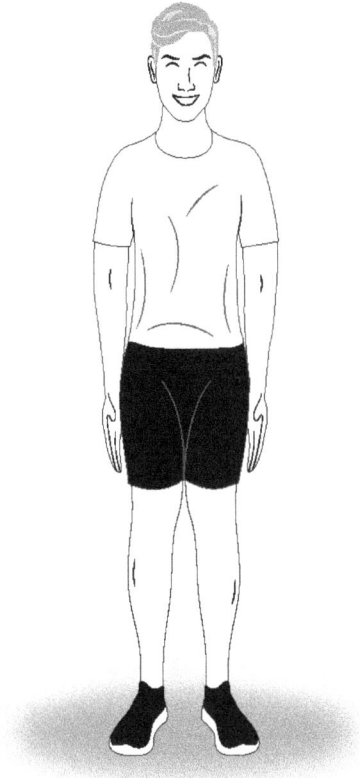

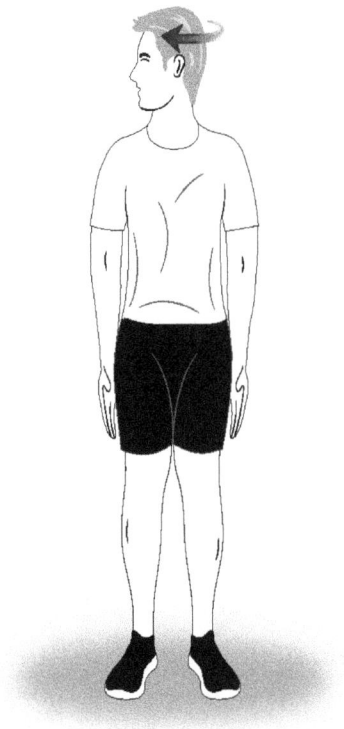

Shoulder Rolls

How This Helps You

How many times a day do you rub your neck or pull up your shoulders, wishing for a moment of relief? If you are like most, probably a lot. We often reach for a cooling gel or other remedies to instantly soothe our pains and discomforts. Even if they help a bit, however, their relief is always short-lived. The good news is that with the shoulder stretches in this chapter, you no longer have to rely on all those over-the-counter remedies to help you alleviate stress, tension, and pain.

Shoulder rolls are one of the stretches that warm up and stretch your muscles, tendons, and joints while increasing the circulation of blood rich in nutrients and oxygen throughout these areas. As a result, shoulders, backs, and necks become less stiff and painful. Additionally, you will notice that as you do the exercise, your shoulders are pulled back and your chest is opened. All these actions, taken together, will substantially help to reduce stress and strain in your neck and shoulder region.

Muscle pain and tightness in the neck and upper back are common symptoms of poor posture. By rolling your shoulders, you loosen and assist your muscles in returning to their correct postural positions. In time, you will develop and maintain a better posture and combat these discomforts.

How to Do It

1. Stand or sit upright, straightening your back to where you still feel comfortable.

2. While maintaining a relaxed posture, slowly push your shoulders forward and raise them toward your ears. Inhale deeply as you raise your shoulders high.

3. As you exhale, squeeze your shoulder blades together, slowly lowering your shoulders back to the starting position. Repeat in continuous circles for a total of 10 times. Start with small circles. As you progress, make your circles larger with smoother and more fluid movements.

4. If that feels comfortable, repeat with 10 circles in the opposite direction.

5. Remember to breathe deeply as you work through these movements, keeping them as smooth, continuous, and complete as you can manage. Ultimately, aspire to make your circles as big as possible while maintaining the fluidity and accuracy of the movement.

Furthermore, as you work through the exercise and those that follow, ensure that you prioritize your own comfort level, physical capability, and safety while remembering to relax during the workout and genuinely enjoy the feeling of your muscles extending and awakening.

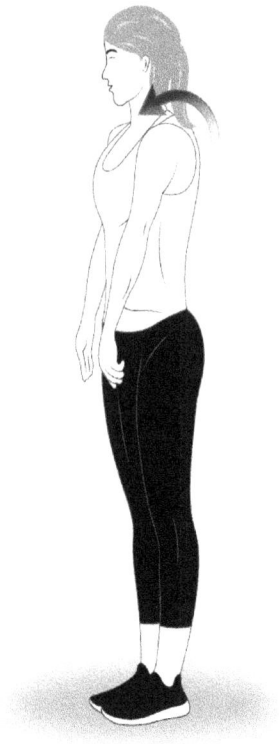

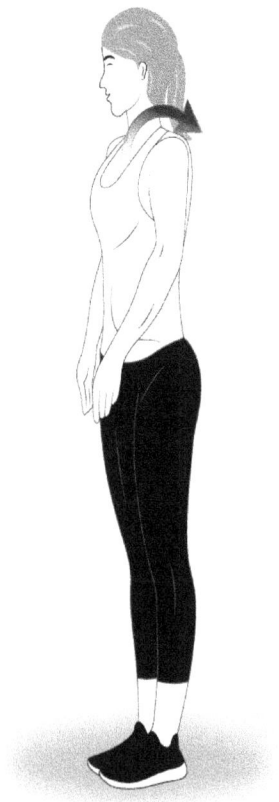

Shoulder Flexion

How This Helps You

Joints become more frictional as we age due to a reduction in synovial fluid. This fluid loss is quite prevalent in our shoulders and arms, which could cause problems in our rotator cuffs (the group of muscles and tendons stabilizing our shoulders). As a result, picking up your laundry basket or fetching a glass from the cupboard can be challenging. Shoulder Flexion exercises are a great way to stretch your shoulder joints and, as a result, allow you a freer range of motion with less pain.

How to Do It

1. Stand tall or sit upright with your arms at your sides and palms facing toward you.

2. Bring your straightened arms out in front of you, then raise them as high as you can while remaining comfortable. Imagine your arms being pulled forward and upward. Feel how your arms and shoulders stretch as your muscles lengthen with each pull.

3. Hold for 5 seconds before returning to your resting position. Repeat for a total of 10 times.

4. Your goal is to point your fingers directly overhead and feel the stretch in your shoulders as your muscles lengthen. As with the other exercises, however, any movement is great as you work toward your goal—as long as you practice good form.

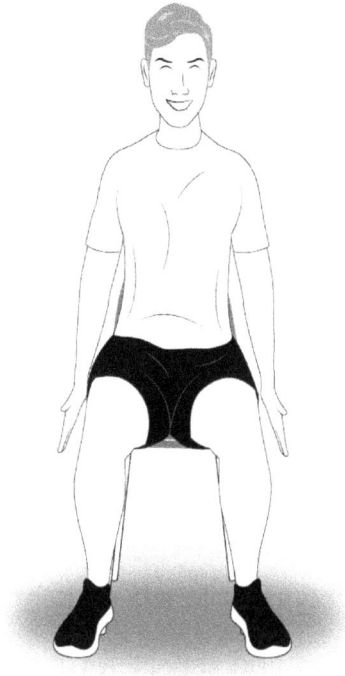

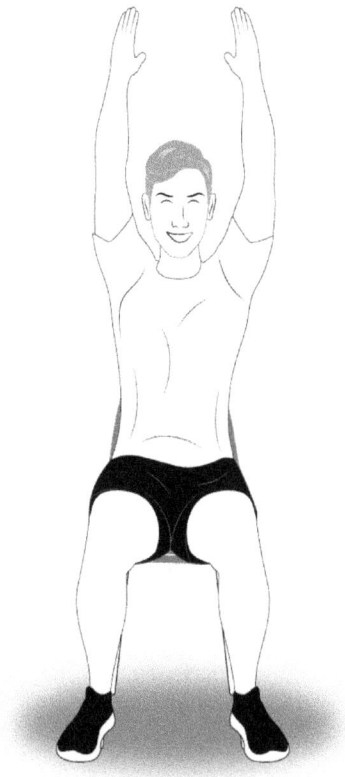

Shoulder Stretch

How This Helps You

We now know that stretching your shoulders improves circulation, posture, and mobility while reducing and preventing injuries, pain, and tightness within these muscles and joints. So, as far as stretching goes, working on your shoulders regularly goes a long way.

How to Do It

1. Stand tall or sit up straight with both arms at your sides.

2. Slowly bring your right arm out in front of you. Keep your arm straight as if you were pointing directly ahead.

3. Using your left arm, slowly bring your right arm toward your body and across your chest while still keeping your right arm straight. Hold for 5 seconds.

4. Remember to breathe deeply, listen to your body, and stretch your shoulder muscles while remaining within your comfort levels and capabilities.

5. Return to your starting position and repeat for a total of 10 times. Do the same with your left shoulder.

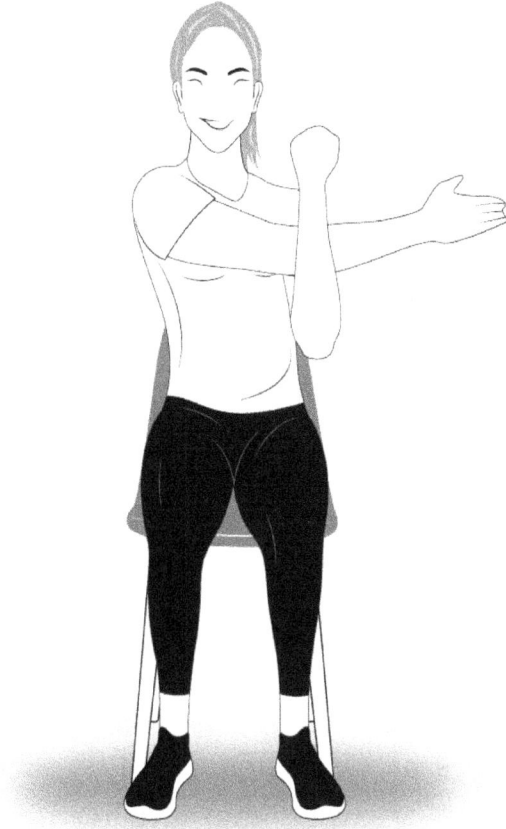

Overhead Stretch

How This Helps You

Oftentimes, we suffer from pain and stiffness in the shoulders, which limits and decreases the range of motion needed to perform overhead-reaching tasks. That is why reaching above your head to grab a bag of bread may feel like a more challenging chore than mopping the floor. This overhead stretch is an excellent way to combat pain, stiffness, and discomfort felt in the shoulders while helping you move with more ease when it comes to reaching. Furthermore, you will benefit from an improved posture, a reduction in respiratory ailments, and a better overall sense of well-being when going about your everyday life.

How to Do It

1. Stand tall or sit up straight with your shoulders relaxed and your head facing forward.

2. Slowly bring both arms up, so your hands are at your ears. Continue raising them past your head, then straighten your arms completely as you reach for the sky.

3. For an even better stretch, attempt this instead: Interlace your fingers before raising your arms upward. Keep your palms facing up as you push them as high as you can while remaining comfortable.

4. Either one of the versions of the stretches will do. Do only the one you are most comfortable with. Do not over-push or injure yourself.

5. Stretch your arms above your head for 5 seconds before slowly lowering them back to the starting position.

6. Repeat for a total of 5 times.

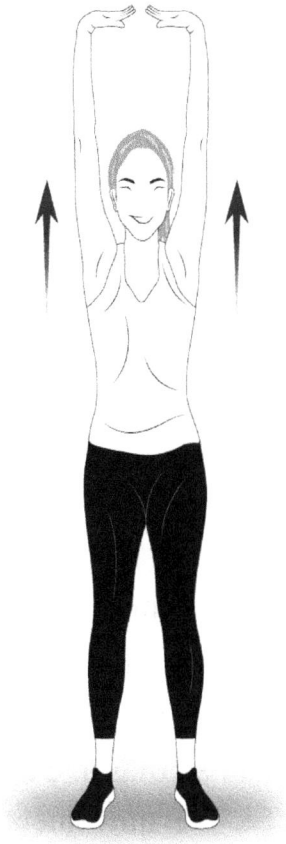

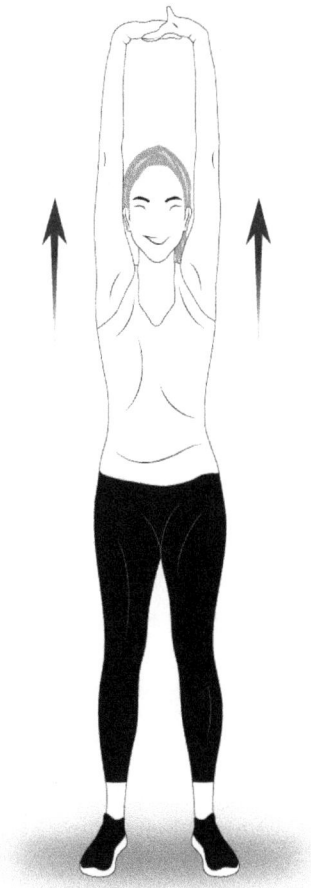

Upper Back Rotation

How This Helps You

Many of us are quite familiar with upper back aches and pains, especially after engaging in activities such as reading or knitting where we tend to hunch over. Moreover, in this day and age where smartphone and computer use is more common, losing good posture to focus on our screens can lead to tightness and pain. By stretching your upper back muscles through rotations, you can relieve and prevent pain, stress, and tension from accumulating over time. Upper Back Rotations will provide you with an improved posture and enhanced overall support so you can continue crafting, reading, or texting to your heart's content!

How to Do It

1. Stand tall or sit up straight with both arms crossed over your chest. Take a deep breath in and out to allow yourself to relax completely.

2. While focusing on keeping your lower body stationary, slowly start rotating your upper body to the right. Remember that twisting like a washing machine at full speed is not the goal here and never should be. The movement from the front to the right should be slow, steady, and gradual.

3. Hold your position for 5 seconds and enjoy the feeling of your upper back muscles stretching. From here, gently return to the starting position and face forward before gradually rotating again, this time to the left, and holding your stretch for another 5 seconds. Remember to exhale slowly into the stretch, and inhale on relaxing.

4. After returning to the starting position again, repeat the rotations a total of 5 times on each side.

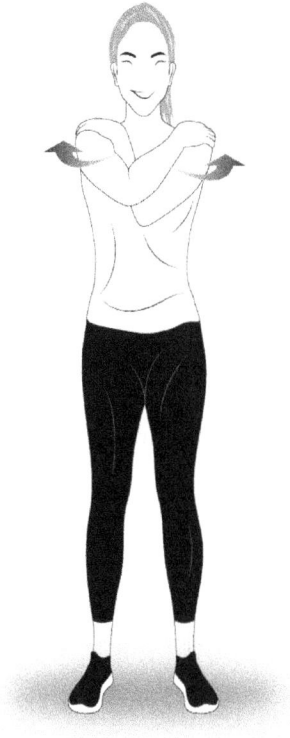

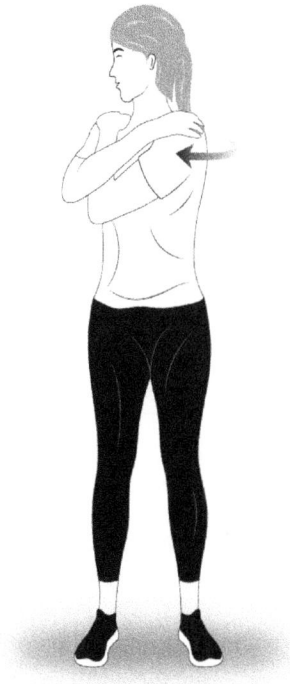

Upper Back Stretch #1

How This Helps You

We often neglect our upper backs, resulting in various problems such as poor posture, limited mobility, rigid muscles, and back aches. If we wish to counteract these hardships and gain the benefits discussed above, we need to stretch these muscles along with those of the chest to ensure that we have enough strength and support to make a change.

How to Do It

1. Stand tall or sit up with your back straightened. Remember to breathe calmly and deeply.

2. Interlace your fingers, if you can, before straightening your arms directly in front of you, palms facing forward.

3. Slowly start pushing your palms toward a focal point in front of you. Imagine that your wrists are bound with rope and that something is gradually pulling on your arms. You should feel your shoulder blades pulling away from one another.

4. Hold this stretch for 5 seconds before relaxing. You should be slowly and deeply exhaling during the stretch, and inhaling when relaxing.

5. Repeat the movement a total of 5 times.

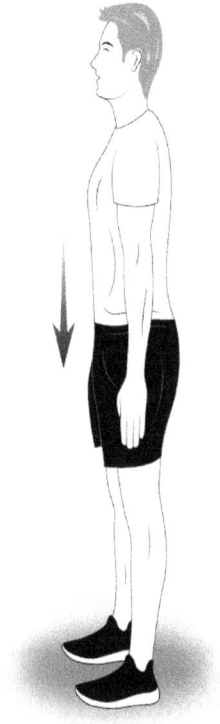

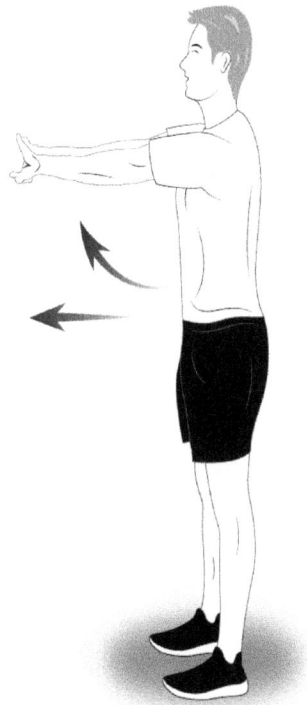

Upper Back Stretch #2

How This Helps You

This exercise holds all the benefits of the two upper-back stretches above. When done regularly, you should experience reduced pain in your upper back, shoulders, and the area around your shoulder blades. The change you will notice with consistency and stretching alone will be astonishing!

How to Do It

1. Sit up straight in a sturdy chair that will remain stationary.

2. Place both hands behind your head, and extend your elbows out and back as far as possible.

3. Gently lean back in the chair, extending yourself over the backrest. If you feel uncomfortable at any given time, lean forward to recuperate before returning to your movement. Allow yourself to truly feel and enjoy the stretch.

4. Hold the stretch for 5 seconds before you return to your starting position.

5. Repeat for a total of 5 times. Remember to breathe slowly and deeply throughout and to keep your comfort in mind at all times.

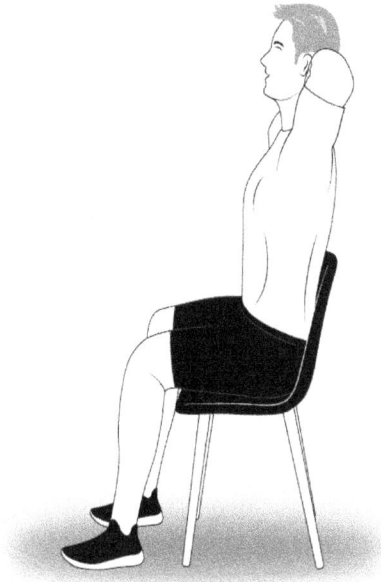

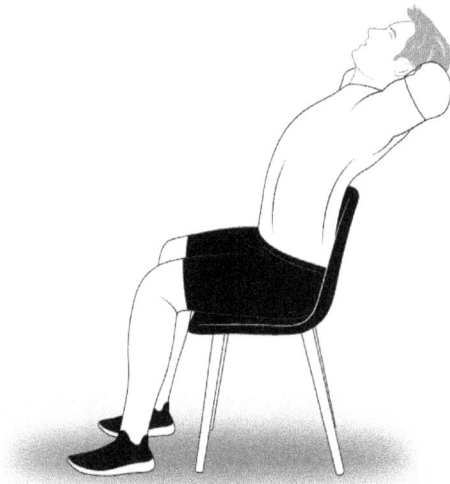

Chest Stretch

How This Helps You

The shoulders, neck, and respiratory system are very often affected by tensed or tight muscles in the chest. You might also find it hard to lift heavy objects or move around without problems as your chest muscles contribute greatly to those actions. In addition to increasing mobility and reducing the risk of muscle injuries, chest stretching stimulates circulation, increases flexibility, improves posture, and facilitates oxygen intake to improve overall breathing comfort. Clearly, your chest muscles are important, and you have to look after them!

How to Do It

1. With your shoulders relaxed, stand tall or sit up straight and focus your gaze straight ahead.

2. Raise your arms directly in front of you and keep them straight and parallel to the ground.

3. Spread your straightened arms apart by stretching them as far back as you can comfortably manage. Imagine that you are an eagle, fully outstretching your wings.

4. As you spread your arms wide, press your shoulder blades together and hold the stretch for 5 seconds before slowly relaxing them again. Exhale into the stretch, and inhale as you relax.

5. Gently bring your arms back in front of you to the starting position.

6. Repeat for a total of 10 times.

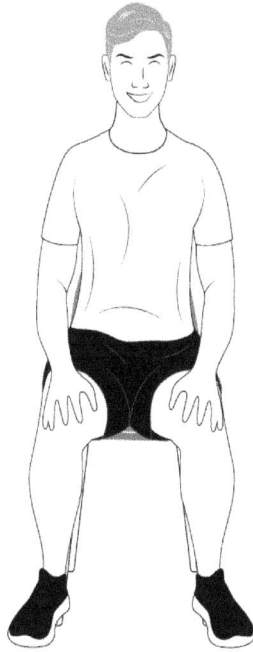

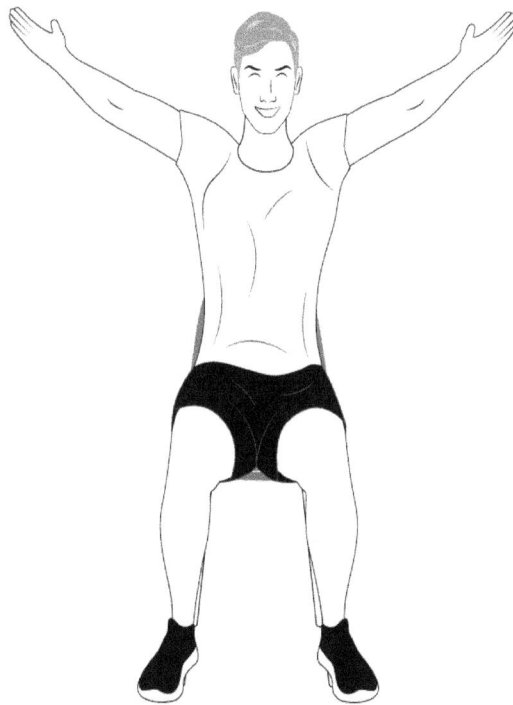

Wrist Extension

How This Helps You

Although you might not have given it much thought, you use your wrist to do a significant number of things: writing, knitting, cooking, doing chores, picking things up, making hand gestures, turning handles, and so on. Therefore, when wrists and arms are sore, stiff, or not as they should be, it is easy to be overcome by a feeling of being less able and independent. With the following stretch, you help increase your range of motion and reduce pain in your wrists, forearms, and elbows so that you are able to do more for longer and without much thought.

How to Do It

1. Stand tall or sit upright. Keep your back straight, shoulders relaxed, and head fixed forward.

2. Slowly bring your right arm out in front of you. Your palm should face forward, and your fingers should point up as if you are directing someone to stop.

3. From there, use your left hand to gently bend your fingers back toward yourself. You should feel the stretch in your wrist, but note how the feeling runs down your forearm. Keep your right arm straightened and hold this position for 5 seconds before letting go.

4. Allow yourself to relax, but keep your arm outstretched. Repeat for a total of 5 times.

5. Lower your arm and return to the starting position, then do the same for the left wrist.

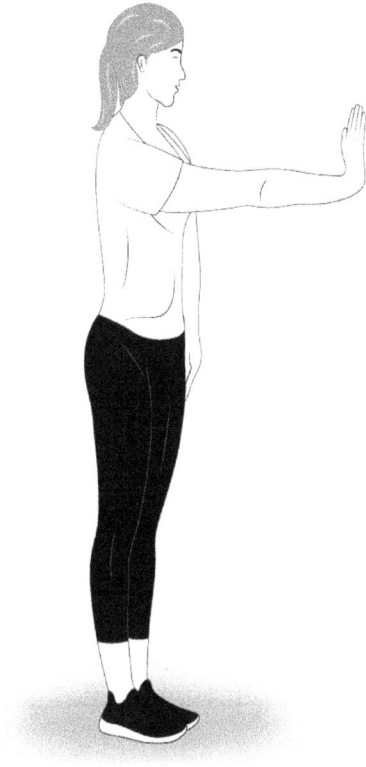
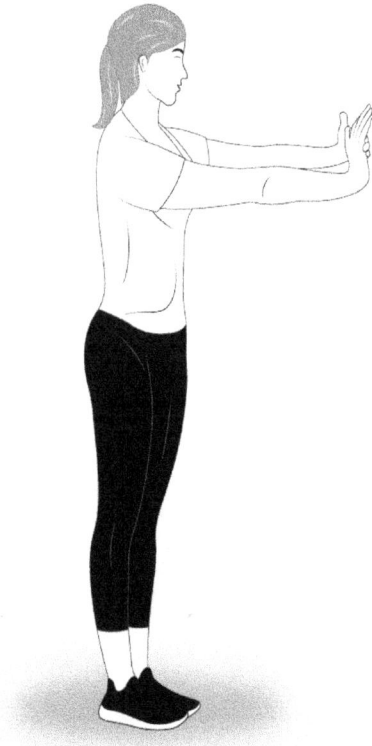

Wrist Flexion

How This Helps You

Along with hand-strengthening exercises, having better mobility and flexibility in your wrist will help you with ordinary activities such as opening jars. It will also improve blood flow and warmth to the muscles, ligaments, and joints while allowing these parts to gain all the oxygen and nutrients they need to function at their best. This wrist exercise, along with the one above, is key in reducing overall pain and tightness while ensuring freedom of the wrist for good!

How to Do It

1. Stand up tall or sit up straight, keeping your shoulders relaxed and your back well-postured.

2. Bring your right arm out directly in front of you and allow your wrist to go limp.

3. Using your left hand, grasp your right fingers and gently bend them toward you. Focus on the muscles in your wrist and forearm; imagine them lengthening and relaxing as you stretch.

4. Hold the stretch for 5 seconds before letting go and allowing yourself to relax, but still holding your arm out in front of you. Repeat for a total of 5 times.

5. When done, return to your resting position before completing the same movements on your left wrist.

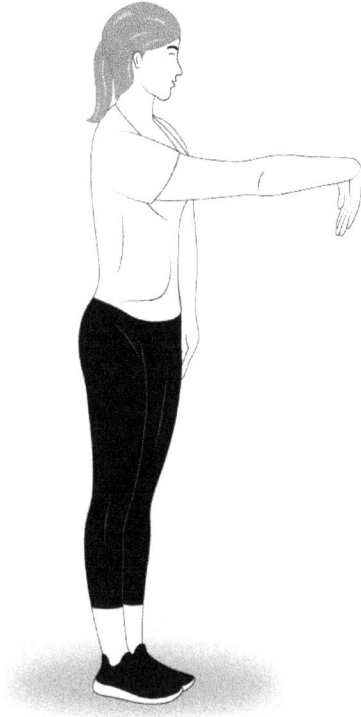

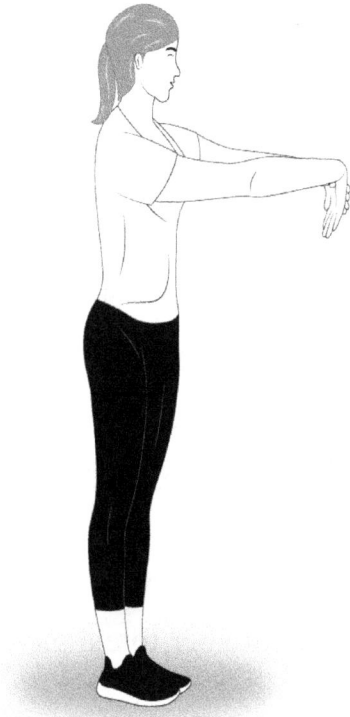

Chapter 5:
Stretching Your Lower Body

Lower Back Forward Flexion

How This Helps You

When you think about it, the lower back is where your upper and lower bodies meet, almost like a bridge between the two. As a bridge and an essential connector, it plays a vital role in supporting your spine and, thus, your overall structural support. Yet, bridges require trusses and support to remain stable. Similarly, your lower back needs strong and healthy muscles to enable them to perform their important function. By stretching this area, you strengthen these muscles and ease the strains, tensions, and pressures often leading to the lower back pain some of us know all too well. Furthermore, you will experience enhanced posture, mobility, and overall sense of motion, all of which will ultimately allow you to support your frame better than ever.

How to Do It

1. Sit up straight in a sturdy, reliable chair that will remain stationary.

2. Slowly bend forward, trying to bring your hands down to your toes. As you do this, feel the natural flex and stretch of your lower back. Do not force the movement. If you cannot touch your toes, simply allow yourself to stretch down as far as you can. You will find yourself being able to reach down further as your flexibility and mobility improve.

3. Hold for 5 seconds as you allow yourself to relax and enjoy the feeling of your muscles stretching.

4. After a good stretch, gradually roll your body up to the starting position.

5. Repeat for a total of 5 times. Remember to exhale as you bend forward and inhale as you sit up.

6. For a more advanced stretch, try this exercise while standing. Move slowly, avoid "bouncing" in and out of the stretch, and do not overdo or force yourself.

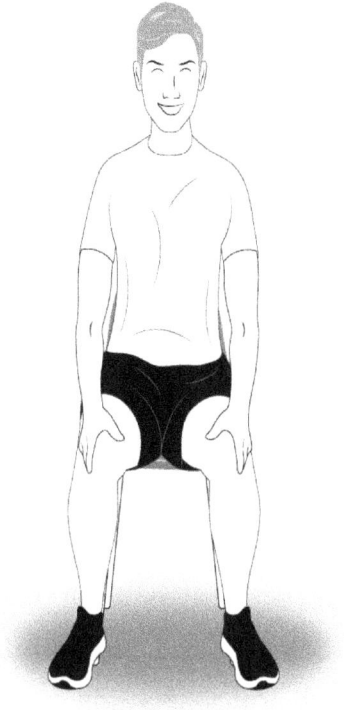

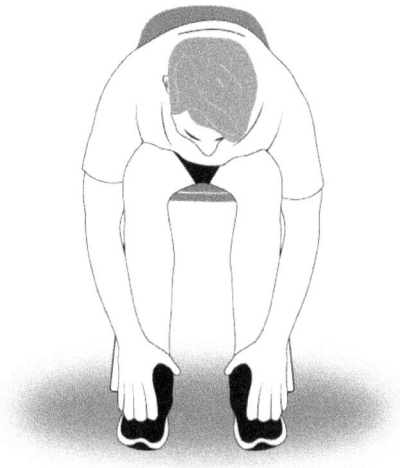

Lower Back Side Flexion

How This Helps You

As with the Forward Flexion stretch above, this Side Flexion exercise supports and improves posture, mobility, and range of motion—all vital to perform various actions including walking and keeping your balance. In short, a good stretch that involves all of your lower back muscles, including those on your side, is remarkably advantageous and will keep you strutting along.

How to Do It

1. Stand tall with your arms hanging down at your sides. If you have difficulty balancing, opt for a reliable and sturdy chair on the side to hold on to.

2. Place your right hand on your right hip. Stretch your left arm upward and extend your fingertips as high as possible.

3. As you exhale, gently bend to your right, moving your left arm overhead with the rest of your body. Hold the stretch for 5 seconds as you feel the left side of your body extend and stretch. Exhale into the stretch.

4. While inhaling, gradually bring your body up to the starting position as you keep your arm above your head.

5. Enjoy this stretch for a total of 10 times, then do the same on the opposite side.

6. When you have completed both sides, note whether one side felt tighter than the other. Understanding how opposite sides of your body feel is one part of how you should listen to and be aware of your physical self. This will help guide you in further exercise sessions as to what areas of your body may need extra attention.

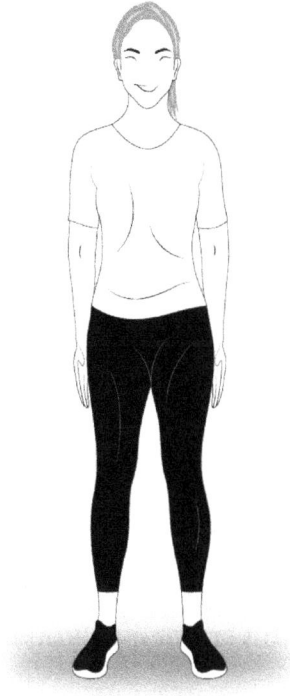

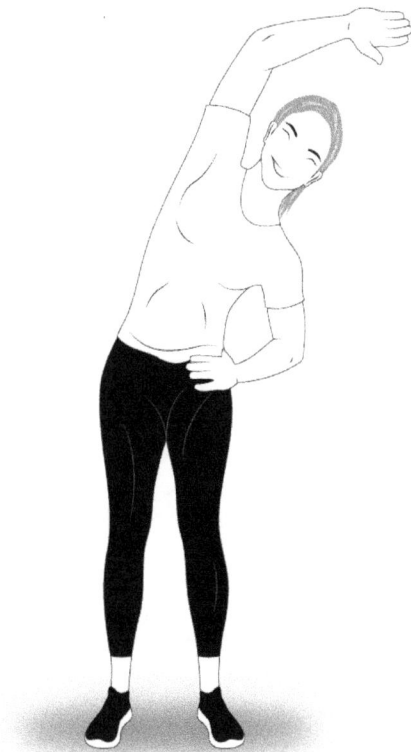

Lower Back Extension

How This Helps You

This stretch can help you improve posture, relieve pain, increase mobility, and prevent back injuries like no other, especially when combined with the strength exercises discussed later in this book. Essentially, therefore, the Lower Back Extension exercise holds the same benefits as the previous two lower back stretches but with an emphasis on injury prevention.

How to Do It

1. Stand tall with your back straight. If possible, stand near something that can offer you support if needed. If you are sitting, choose a sturdy, stable chair, and sit towards the front of your seat.

2. Place both palms on your lower back, fingers pointing down.

3. With your hands in place, exhale deeply as you gradually start leaning backward, pushing your hands into your lower back as you do so.

4. Hold for 5 seconds and allow yourself to enjoy the feeling of your lower back muscles expanding.

5. If at any time you feel yourself losing balance, use your support to assist you. Take a moment to regain your balance and footing before resuming the exercise.

6. Slowly move back to your starting position as you inhale and relax.

7. Repeat for a total of 5 times.

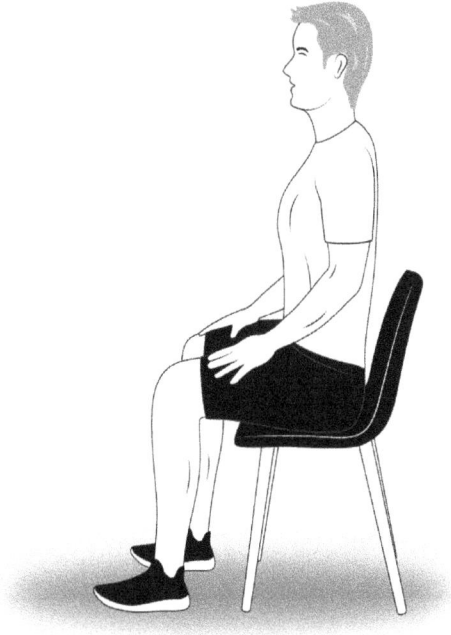

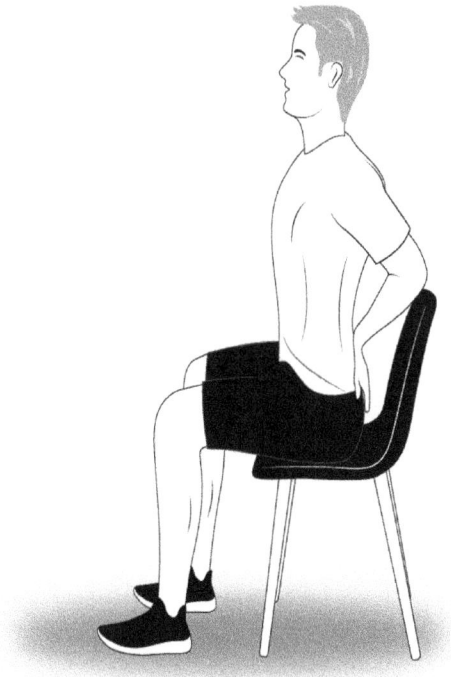

Hip Flexion

How This Helps You

Tight and tense gluteal or buttock muscles are prominent contributors to lower body pain. Fortunately, this stretch is a great way to reduce these discomforts while promoting better lower body movements when walking, standing, and sitting.

How to Do It

1. Sit up straight on the front portion of a sturdy, reliable chair. You can also lie down with your back flat on the floor.

2. Lift your right knee up towards you and into both of your hands.

3. Exhale and gently pull your right leg toward your body as much as you comfortably can.

4. Hold for 5 seconds. Feel the stretch in your buttock and hip muscles as you hug your knee.

5. Relax your muscles as you release the stretch while inhaling, then repeat for a total of 5 times.

6. Do the same with your left side.

7. As you progress, you can also try doing this stretch with both legs simultaneously.

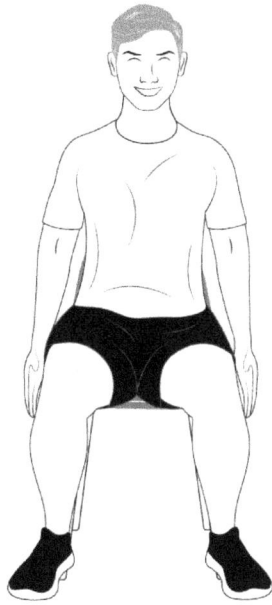

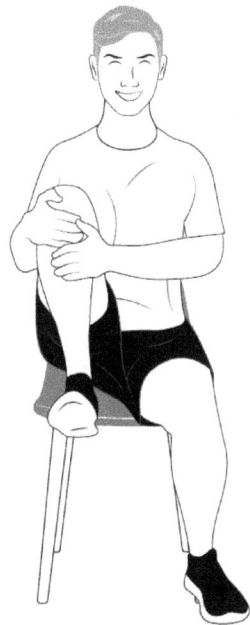

Piriformis Stretch

How This Helps You

The piriformis is a peculiar-sounding muscle in the gluteal or buttock region. This flat, narrow muscle runs from the lower spine through the hips, buttocks, and thighs, aiding us in almost every movement we make. This stretch will help loosen and lengthen these muscles while improving the strength and mobility of the piriformis and the surrounding hip and buttock muscles. For many people, this exercise will help relieve the pain and symptoms associated with *sciatic neuritis (nerve)* and piriformis syndrome. These are common conditions and disorders affecting the piriformis and the sciatic nerves, which are responsible for the lower body's motor and sensory functioning. Therefore, keeping your piriformis in prime condition means less pain and freer movement for much of your lower body.

How to Do It

1. Sit up straight on the front portion of your chair or lie with your back flat on the floor.

2. Bring your right ankle up to rest on your left knee. If getting your ankle up that far is too difficult while seated, don't be discouraged. It's fine to lower your left knee to meet your right ankle.

3. Slowly start pressing down on your right knee as you gently bend forward. Try keeping your posture as upright as possible and avoid arching your back. If you're lying on the floor, bring your left knee toward your body as you feel your right piriformis stretch.

4. Hold for 5 seconds as you exhale. You will feel a remarkable stretch and pulling sensation in your hip, buttock, and piriformis regions. Enjoy this feeling!

5. After holding your stretch, relax as you inhale and return to your starting position. Repeat for a total of 5 times.

6. When you are done, treat your opposite side to the same great stretch.

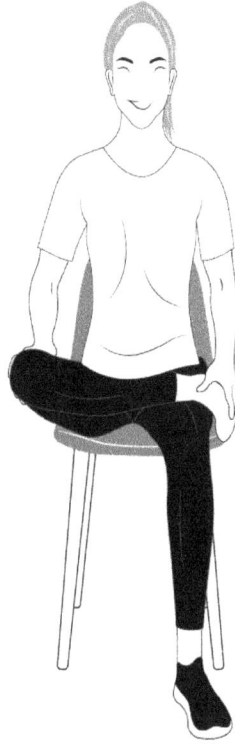

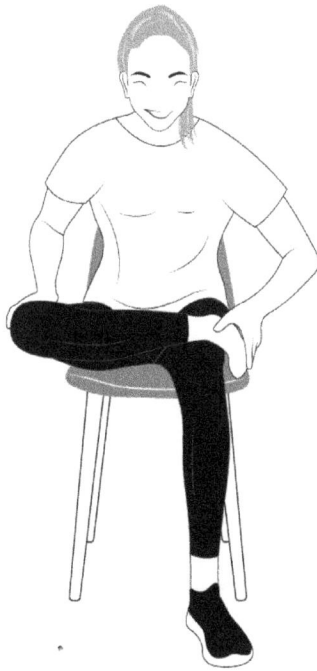

Hamstring Stretch

How This Helps You

The muscles that run along the back of your thigh (called hamstrings) make it possible for you to extend your leg behind you, bend your knee, and provide support as you walk or run. By stretching your hamstrings, you ease these muscles while keeping them strong, healthy, and flexible. This will improve your stance and relieve you from pains such as those in the lower back and feet. Furthermore, you will find that leaning forward and reaching down to grab your shoes will become much easier to do.

How to Do It

1. Stand straight with your chair on your right side for balance and support. If you cannot stand, take a seat on the front portion of your chair.

2. Take a step back with your right leg while keeping the left leg straight. The toes of both feet should be pointing forward. If you are sitting, stretch your left leg out straight in front of you while your right foot takes a step back.

3. Keep your back straight as you slowly bend forward, using the chair to support you when needed. You should feel the back of your left thigh stretching and lengthening as you are doing so. Lean forward only as far as you comfortably can while giving yourself a nice stretch. Do not force the stretch; do it gently and smoothly, like tugging on a rubber band.

4. Repeat the stretch a total of 5 times before bringing your right leg back to the starting position.

5. Duplicate the exercise with your right hamstring by moving the chair to your left side and taking your left leg back. If you are sitting, extend your right leg out in front of you as your left leg moves back.

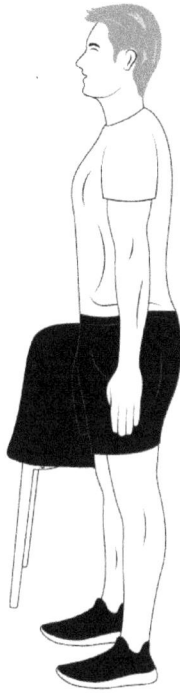

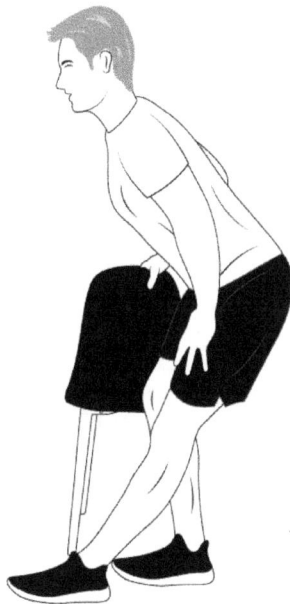

Inner Thigh Stretch

How This Helps You

The inner thighs, or adductors, are essential in keeping us balanced, stable, and moving around safely, comfortably, and without any injuries. Stretching your inner thighs allows you to maintain this stability, specifically affecting your hips, knees, lower back, and core while easing tension in the legs and groin. The front, back, and lateral muscles of your thighs work in concert with each other. Paying attention to the often-neglected adductors will help to ensure a balanced and comprehensive improvement in your entire thigh area.

How to Do It

1. Stand tall with a chair in front of you for balance and support. If you are unable to stand, sit on the front portion of your chair.

2. Take a step to the side with your right leg; your toes should point to the side. If seated, keep your right leg out to the side with your toes pointing straight ahead of you.

3. Slowly bend your left knee, holding onto the chair for balance if needed. If you are sitting comfortably, start leaning forward. If you feel uncomfortable or lose your balance, there is no need to worry. Simply reset yourself and try again. You can do it! Remember that even a small movement with this exercise will help to elongate your adductors.

4. Hold each stretch for 5 seconds as you experience the lengthening of your entire inner thigh area. For many people, this will be the first time that they realize how tight they are in that area.

5. After 5 nice stretches, return to your starting position, then do the same on your opposite side.

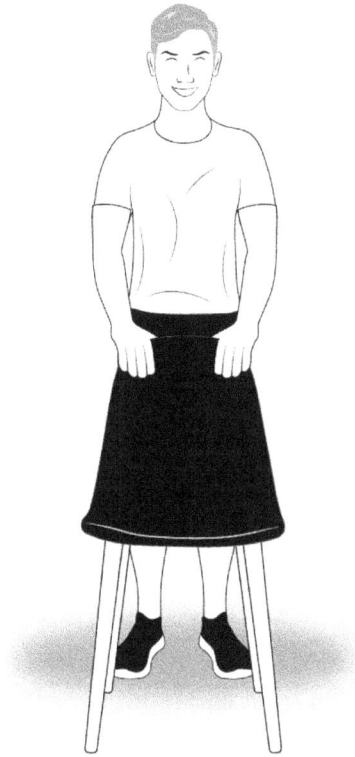

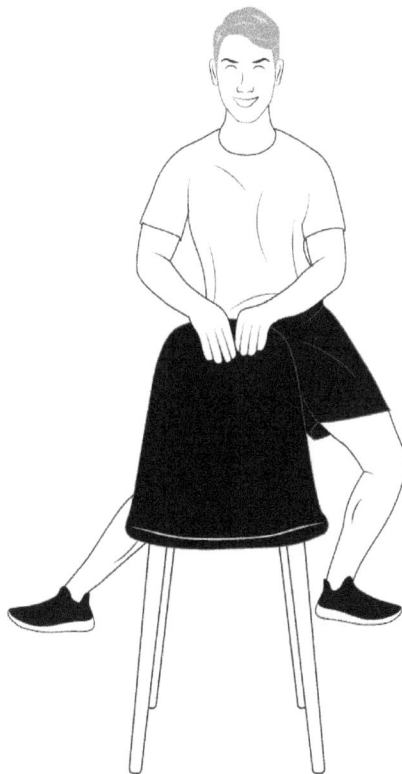

Quadriceps Stretch

How This Helps You

The muscles in the front of your thighs, sometimes called quadriceps or quads, are a major muscle group that allows you to perform a variety of movements such as kicking, jumping, and walking. They absorb the force of your feet hitting the ground, regulate your walk, and keep you moving more steadily. By stretching these muscles, you improve circulation to the quads which, in turn, reduces tension and stiffness, aids mobility, enhances performance, and strengthens and stabilizes the knees. It will also assist in reducing any aches and pains in the lower back, knees, and thighs.

How to Do It

1. Stand tall behind your chair, using it for balance and support.

2. Keep your left leg stable and straight as you bend your right leg enough to grab onto your feet with your right hand. If you cannot clutch onto your foot, start by grabbing your ankle or using a small towel or resistance band to pull your foot or ankle toward you. Slow, steady, and safe are the key guidelines to remember here.

3. Continue bending the right leg as far and as much as you comfortably can. As your leg is bent, get as much of a good stretch on the front of your thigh as you comfortably can. Do not fight the stretch, but instead, allow your muscles to lengthen.

4. Hold the stretch for 5 seconds, then return to your starting position.

5. Repeat the stretch a total of 5 times. Get a sense of how your quadriceps have already loosened from your first stretch to your fifth.

6. Now treat your left quad to the same five stretches.

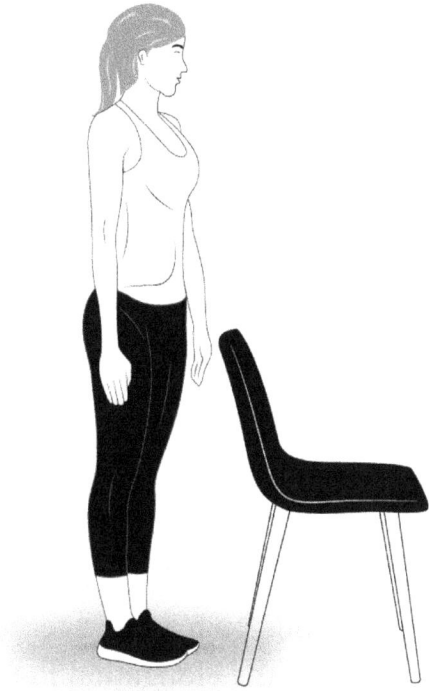
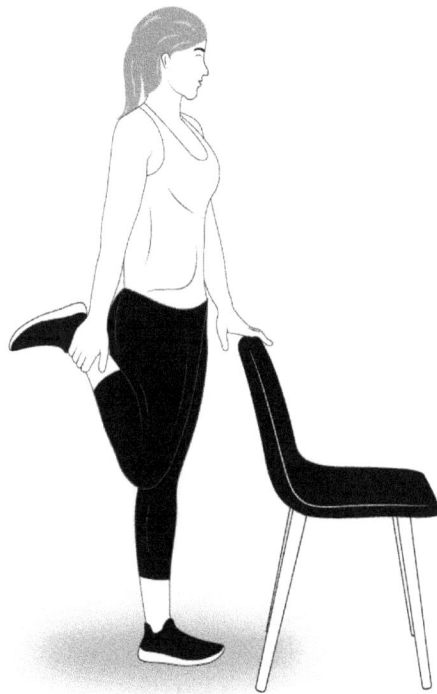

Calf Stretch

How This Helps You

Your calves are involved in many of the activities we do every day, such as walking and standing. Therefore, when they are tight and tense, it can be hard to get around. Accompanying pain in the foot, leg, and knee is common as well. By stretching these muscles, you activate them, stimulate blood flow, and allow yourself a better range of motion and flexibility while avoiding injuries. Sooner or later, you will not mind standing in line at the mall—although we cannot do much about how long you will have to wait.

How to Do It

1. Stand behind a sturdy chair with both hands resting on top of the backrest.

2. Take a step back with your right foot, toes pointing forward.

3. Bend your left knee while keeping both your heels on the floor. As you continue bending your left knee further, feel the elongation in your right calf muscle and allow all that tension to be released.

4. Hold for 5 seconds before returning to the starting position.

5. Repeat for a total of 5 times before stretching your left calf.

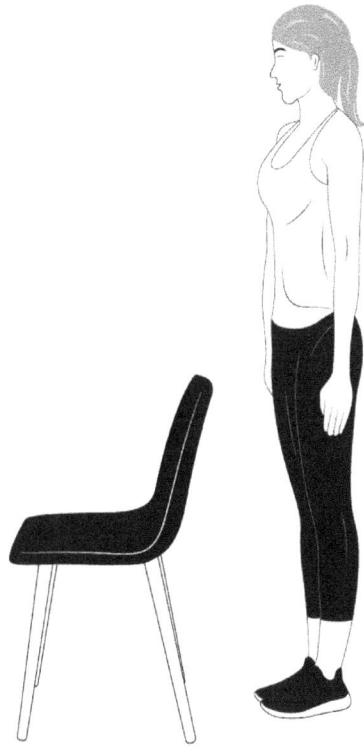

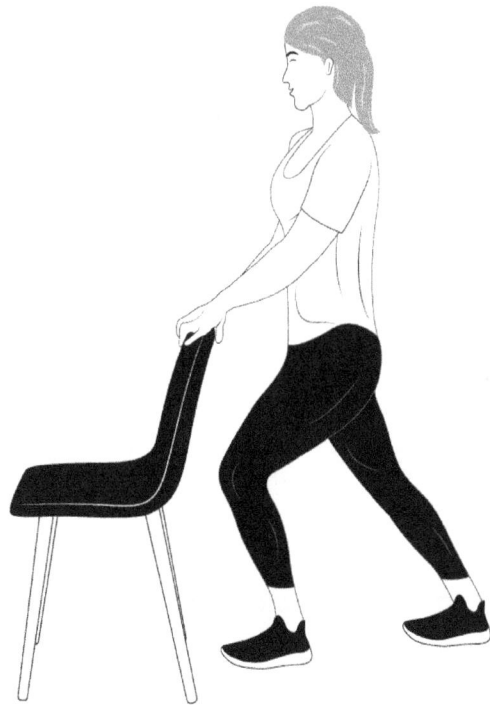

Chapter 6:
Why Is Muscle Strength Important?

As I was thinking about the importance of strong muscles, my mind drifted to a cartoon image I once saw. It was of a man thoroughly covered in orthopedic casts from head to toe. In fact, the only visible part of him were his two oval eyes. Clearly, he was in much distress and pain, and his casts certainly made him unable to move. Whatever the cause of his injuries and the resulting casts, he was surely going to be stuck in bed and immobile for quite some time.

I mention that image to you as I reflect on the fact that unused and immobile muscles lose their tone and strength over time, a process commonly known as atrophy. That is the bad news. The really good news, however, is that muscle tone and strength can be regained. The human body is amazing in that way! In many ways, actually. Nature allows us to help ourselves, quite literally, get back on our own feet simply by using, working, and conditioning our bodies and returning to our healthier selves. Muscles do not disappear when they are not used; they just need to be put back into motion like a rusty bike that needs some oiling.

Hopefully, you are not in a full-body cast rendering you unable to move. There are other reasons, however, that may lead to muscle atrophy in varying degrees whether the cause is an illness, a sedentary lifestyle, pain, or even something as simple as not knowing how to exercise properly. Without use, muscles weaken and become less able to complete the movements and tasks that we need to accomplish in life.

As I mentioned above, the great thing about muscles is that we can take steps to rebuild strength, reclaim good tone, and reverse the atrophy that may now exist. If you take care of your muscles, they will take care of you. If you help your muscles stay in prime condition, they will be there for you to perform any of the myriad tasks that you face each day. If, in your mind, you want to unload groceries from the car but you fear that your body cannot do so, it will only lead to frustration and a loss of independence. This is why people often say that your mind and body have to be in tune. They rely on and work with each other to keep you humming through your daily activities.

The takeaway here is that even if you have not been exercising and have lost the muscle tone and strength you used to have, it is not a lost cause. Slowly, with time and repetition, you can rebuild your strength, improve body mechanics, and happily regain all of the benefits that your body can provide for your active life.

The Benefits of Strengthening Your Muscles

Toning and strengthening our muscles, and keeping them that way, are necessary for us to carry on with our lives. The strength of our muscles affects everything from simple activities of daily living such as getting up from the sofa or preparing dinner, to enjoy the world around us with a pleasant hike in the woods.

You likely already know many of these benefits, such as these:

- **Weight management**: We know that an above-average weight or a high amount of fat within the body is detrimental to our health. It can cause varied conditions, diseases, and threats to your body, health, and overall quality of life. Strength training is an excellent way to shed some pounds and keep them off for good. It increases the metabolism by building muscle mass and allowing the metabolism to stay active hours after you have completed your workout. This means that calories are burned and used more efficiently, and you have more muscles to help your health. Fat and added weight are shredded and better managed, and your life is left feeling lighter and better than ever! Coupled with a sensible diet, strengthening your muscles will quicken your path toward your weight loss goals.

- **Develops stronger bones**: Strength training is essential for bone development and ensuring they are protected and healthy. With strength training, stress is temporarily placed on the bones. This pressure on the bones triggers them to respond by rebuilding their strength. As a result, bone density increases, and the risk of developing bone diseases and conditions such as osteoporosis is reduced. Moreover, when the muscles connected to our bones contract, they stimulate the cells within our bones to produce more proteins and transport more minerals to them, thereby increasing their overall mineral density. Bones are left stronger, denser, and healthier.

- **Manages and prevents diseases and chronic conditions**: Strength training, like all exercises, keeps you healthy and reduces your chance of developing various diseases while helping you control the signs and symptoms of those you may already have. Strength training helps reduce abdominal fat, blood pressure, and high cholesterol while improving circulation and the strength of the heart and blood vessels. This means that you also have a lower risk of developing heart disease. Moreover, it helps your body more effectively remove glucose from the body, which helps manage blood sugar levels and symptoms of diabetes while reducing your risk of developing the condition in the first place. Your health will be in good hands as your body's ability to prevent, manage, and sometimes overcome diseases will help you thrive and improve.

- **Building stronger, healthier muscle mass**: The goal of resistance training is to challenge your muscles to resist an opposing force, such as weights, bands, or even your own body weight. As a result, muscles work and contract to increase their strength, tone, endurance, and power. Muscles must be strong, sturdy, and stable for our bones to be protected and cared for, our muscles to be healthy, and our balance and coordination to be maintained. In short, muscles are critical to keeping our health at its best and improving some of the more unhealthy gaps we have. They can help us do just that through strength training.

- **Prevents falls and protects against injuries**: Strength training supports and improves your balance, coordination, posture, flexibility, range of motion, and overall mobility. Taking care of these aspects is crucial for ensuring that your body is well supported. This allows you to prevent falls more effectively. If you do happen to fall, you may reduce the severity of injuries and consequences due to the body's ability to recover and heal faster. It can also provide additional support, protection, recovery, and care against injuries beyond falls, such as during an exercise, cleaning your home, or lifting heavy items. By reinforcing your joints through strength training, your bones become more robust, your muscles firm up, your body mechanics improve, and injuries are more effectively prevented and managed.

- **Improves brain health**: As we engage in strength training, blood and nutrients circulating throughout our body, including in our brain, are dispersed more effectively and in greater quantities, while inflammation is reduced or avoided. This means that resistance training can improve brain health and power, heighten cognitive functioning, and even prevent and protect us against age-related cognitive decline. It has also been shown to reduce symptoms of mental disorders such as clinical depression and anxiety while regulating and boosting one's mood through managing stress and releasing endorphins. Strength training may also improve sleep patterns and quality, allowing you to wake up with more energy.

The quick list above are only a few of the benefits you can gain from engaging in strength training and accepting it as part of your everyday life. You will find that you are more powerful and better able to perform daily tasks such as carrying groceries, playing sports, completing your chores, and more. Your overall quality of life will show significant improvements, and with each passing day you will find yourself feeling healthier and happier.

Chapter 7:
Upper Body Strength Exercises

Push-up

How This Helps You

In addition to targeting the shoulders, arms, chest, back, stomach, hips, and wrists, push-ups are easy and convenient for most people to perform. This common exercise supports bone strength and, thus, overall bone health. As you can see, push-ups primarily focus on the upper body, which is utilized for a variety of activities, including picking things up, pushing and moving them around, and even bracing ourselves if we trip and stumble. Furthermore, your core strength will increase, your posture will improve, your heart will be healthier, and your functional fitness will get a boost. You will find it easier to carry out your daily activities with more stability and vibrancy.

How to Do It

1. Stand about an arm's length away from a stable, flat surface, such as a wall or the back of a stationary chair. For the purpose of this exercise, I will use a wall as an example.

2. Spread your feet so they are shoulder-width apart. Keep your toes pointing forward.

3. Place both palms on the wall with your fingers pointing upwards.

4. Slowly bend your elbows as you bring your chest forward to the wall, just shy of touching it.

5. Next, straighten your arms as you push yourself away from the wall and back to your starting position. Inhale as you move towards the wall, and exhale as you push away.

6. Feel your muscles working as you move closer to the wall as well as when you push away. Make every movement count!

7. Repeat this a total of 10 times before returning to the starting position. Feel free to take breaks between each repetition as you deem necessary.

8. As you advance, you can attempt the same exercise but vary the space between your palms: Spread your arms wider, bring them closer, or place them directly in front of

you. You will feel different portions of your chest being worked. Another advanced variation you can try as you progress is slightly increasing the distance between you and the wall. Ultimately, if you excel at that, try using the floor rather than the wall.

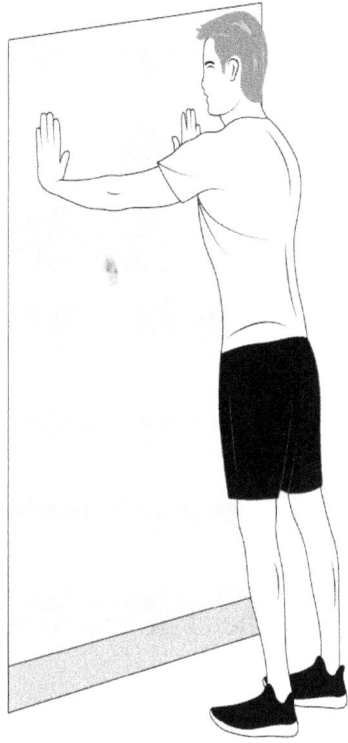

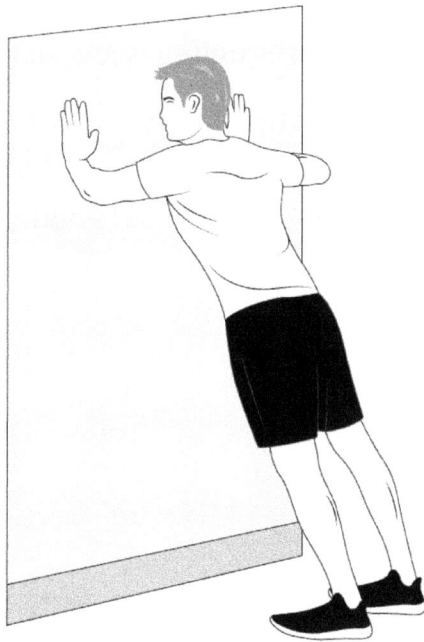

Standing Row

How This Helps You

"Rowing" is a superb exercise for your overall fitness and strength. It is a low-impact, natural movement that strengthens the upper body. It helps strengthen the heart, expands the lungs, elevates your mood, demands minimal stress, and aids you in preventing falls and other injuries. You will strengthen and condition major muscle groups just as oarsmen do!

How to Do It

1. Position yourself approximately an arm's length behind the back of a stationary chair. For balance, hold your left hand on the chair's back while keeping your right arm relaxed at your side.

2. Keep your back straight and your head in line with your back as you bend forward at 45 degrees.

3. Now, bend your right elbow and pull your right arm back until you can squeeze your right shoulder blade. Move as smoothly and thoroughly as you can without jerking. Remember to exhale as you contract your muscles and inhale once you relax them.

4. Hold your contraction for 3 seconds before you relax.

5. Repeat for a total of 10 times before rowing with your left arm.

6. Once you master the exercise described, you can try holding onto a weight with your moving arm. If you do not have dumbbells or kettlebells at home, you can use alternatives such as a filled water bottle, canned goods, or even packets of rice or beans.

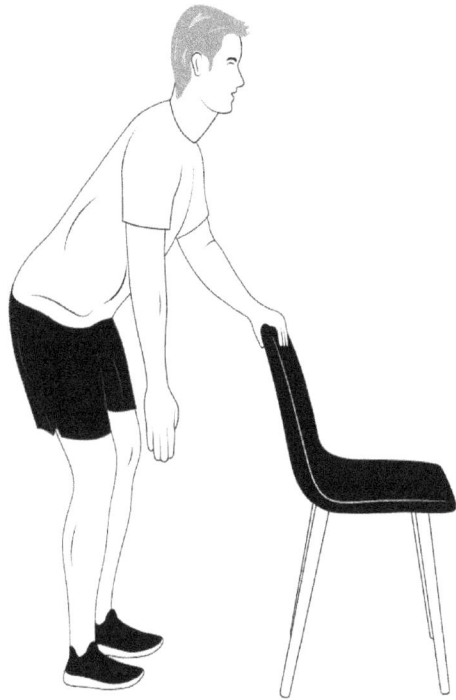

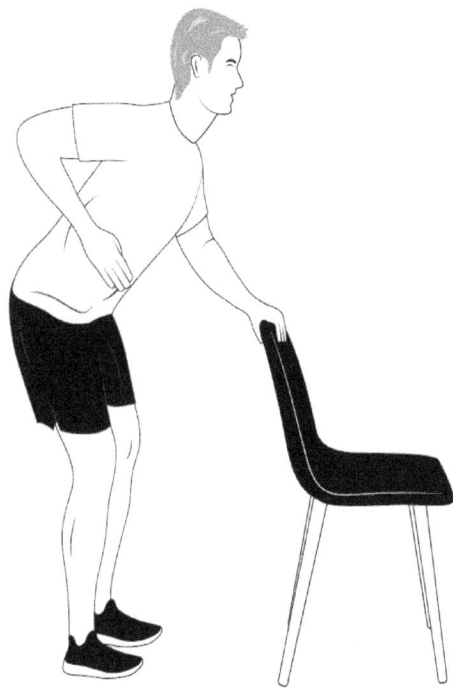

Seated Row

How This Helps You

The benefits of a seated row are much like those you will get from the Standing Row exercise above. Although seated, doing the movements slowly and comprehensively will ensure the same improvements to your heart, lungs, arms, back, and shoulders. Overall, the exercise will aid you in improving your posture, balance, strength, and general health.

How to Do It

1. Sit tall in your chair with both feet flat on the ground, chest up, and eyes fixed forward. Remember to keep your posture in mind throughout the exercise.

2. Slowly bend forward at a 45-degree angle with both hands on your thighs.

3. Lift your right arm in front of you with your palm facing inward. Keep your left arm relaxed on your thigh.

4. Gradually bring your right elbow back as far as possible until you feel your shoulder blade contracting. Stay comfortable and enjoy this feeling.

5. Relax by straightening your right arm out in front of you.

6. Repeat for a total of 10 times before rowing with your left arm.

7. As you master the exercise and advance, use weights in your hands to provide you with a greater challenge.

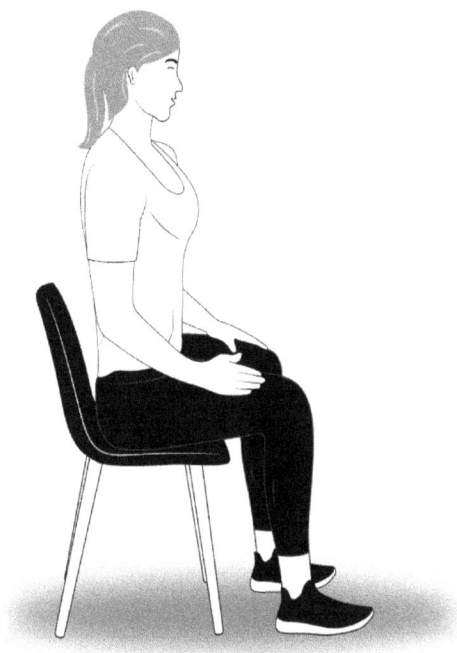

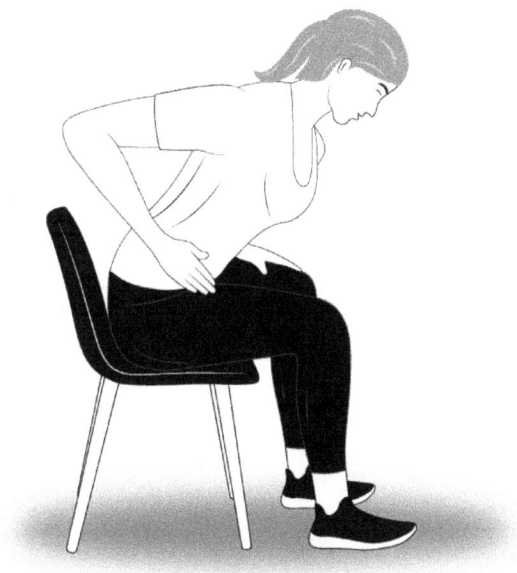

Shoulder Press

How This Helps You

This exercise stimulates and benefits more than just the muscles in your shoulders, arms, torso, and back. Pressure and work placed on the bones cause them to grow stronger and denser, which decreases the likelihood of osteoporosis or at least manages its effects. This means less pain and more range of motion. Further, when your bones and muscles grow more robust, you are better equipped to stabilize and balance the body. This can result in fewer injuries and a more effective undertaking of daily activities.

How to Do It

1. Sit tall in your chair, look straight ahead, and keep both feet planted on the ground.

2. Remember to maintain a proper posture throughout the exercise as this will allow you to get the most out of the exercise.

3. Slowly bring both arms to your shoulders with your palms facing one another.

4. From there, raise your arms up, reaching for the ceiling or sky as far as possible. Do not force the movement past your level of comfortability; always keep your safety in mind.

5. Return your arms down to your shoulders.

6. Repeat for a total of 10 times.

7. As you advance and master the exercise, you can add light weights to your lift. Feel free to challenge yourself, but do not overdo it or use weights that are too heavy to handle. It is far better to maintain proper form.

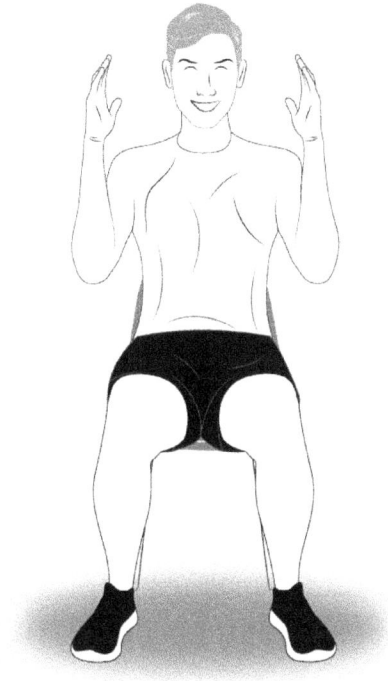

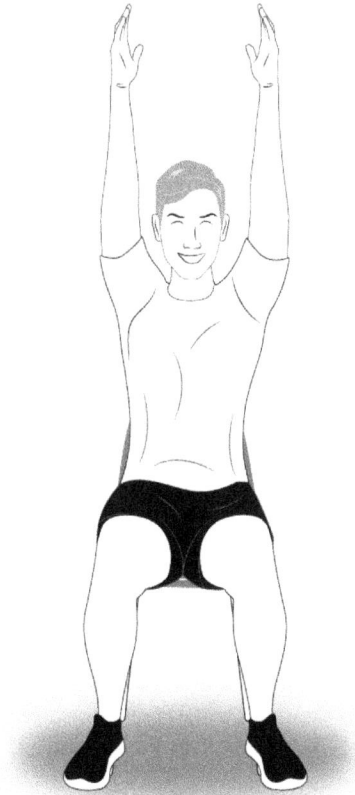

Shoulder Forward Raise

How This Helps You

Shoulder Forward Raises are primarily beneficial for your shoulders, although they also target and work other muscles such as your chest, upper back, and arms. You should see improvements in the size, strength, stability, and mobility of your shoulders, which will help you lift and carry things around. You might also note that exercises requiring your shoulders are easier to perform which will, in turn, assist and enhance your ability to increase your weights and repetitions. There will be less strain and more ease in your everyday life.

How to Do It

1. Sit tall in your chair with both of your feet on the ground.

2. Keep your arms at your sides, palms facing toward you.

3. Straighten your arms as you bring them forward and raise them high in front of you. Once you are at the top of your movement, hold for 2 seconds. Remember to look straight ahead and maintain good posture as you feel the muscles in your shoulders work.

4. Gradually return your arms to your sides. Remember that the movement returning to your resting position is just as important as raising them.

5. Repeat for a total of 10 times.

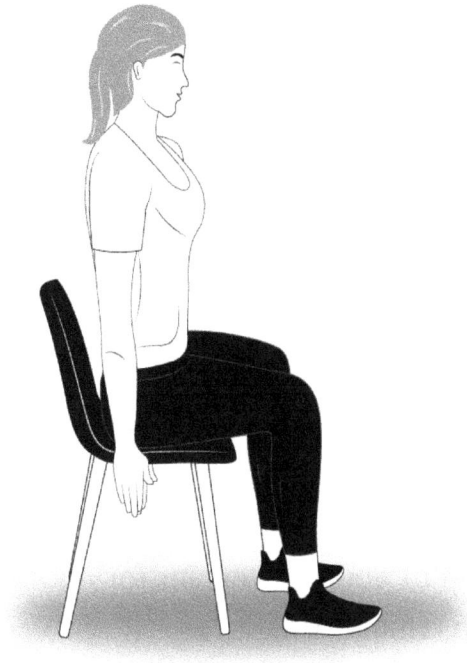
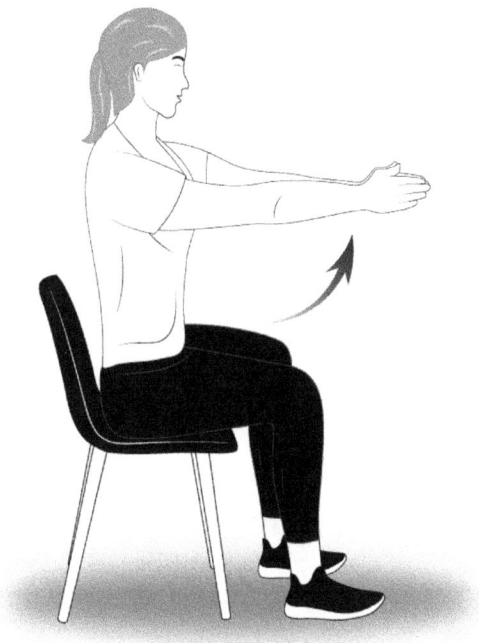

Shoulder Lateral Raise

How This Helps You

Shoulder Lateral Raises help build and strengthen muscles in the shoulders and surrounding areas such as the upper back, arms, and neck. You should notice increased mobility in these areas which will aid you in several daily activities and help you live more freely.

How to Do It

1. Stand or sit tall with your hands by your sides and palms facing toward you.

2. Keep both arms straight yet relaxed as you use your lateral or side shoulder muscles to lift your arms up, making a T-shape with your frame and holding your arms parallel to the ground.

3. Hold your pose at the top of your movement for two seconds. Avoid "flapping" your arms up and down; try to remain still.

4. Return to your starting position by slowly lowering your arms down to your sides.

5. Repeat for a total of 10 times.

6. As with many exercises in the book, feel free to employ the use of weights when you feel you are ready to progress.

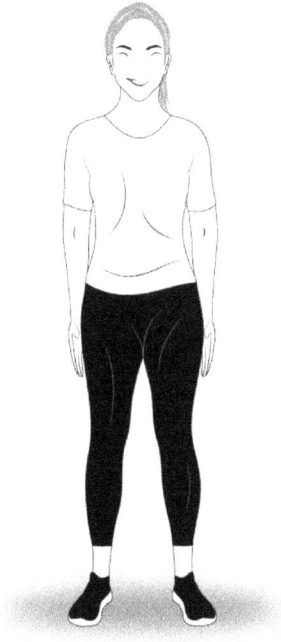

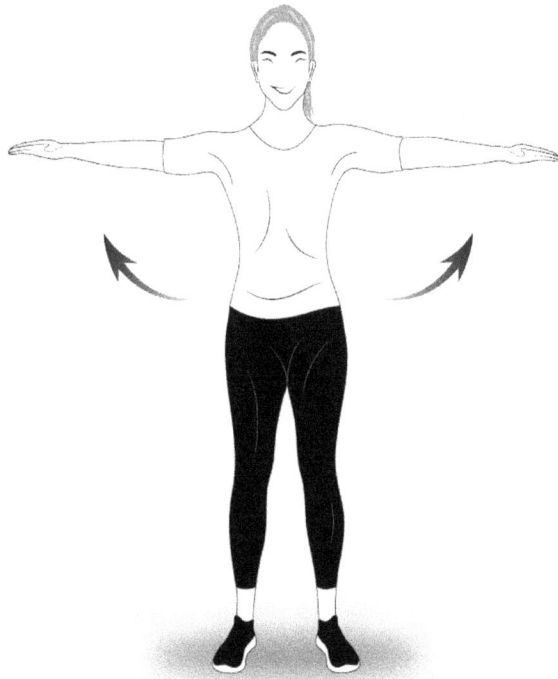

Scapula Squeeze

How This Helps You

Scapulas, or shoulder blades, play an integral role in the smooth movement of the upper extremities. Therefore, the importance of keeping them strong and working adequately should come as no surprise. This exercise will ably improve your posture, especially if you tend to "round" your shoulders forward. By stabilizing your scapulas, you activate your upper limbs and neck muscles, which helps you realign your frame. Strengthening your upper back muscles further stabilizes your shoulders and upper limbs. The results will be evident in increased ease with tasks involving pushing, pulling, and holding onto items.

How to Do It

1. Sit straight in your chair with both hands on your hips. Keep your shoulders down.

2. Inhale, then exhale as you gradually move your elbows back and squeeze your shoulder blades together.

3. Hold the compression for 3 seconds before easing back into your starting position. Remember to inhale as you return.

4. Repeat for a total of 10 times.

5. Keep your hands fixed on your hips throughout the exercise, and ensure that your back is straight. Your movements and transitioning between moves should be slow, sure, and comfortable.

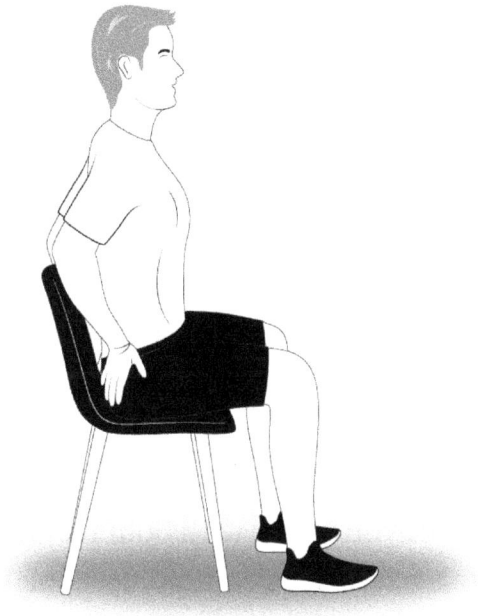

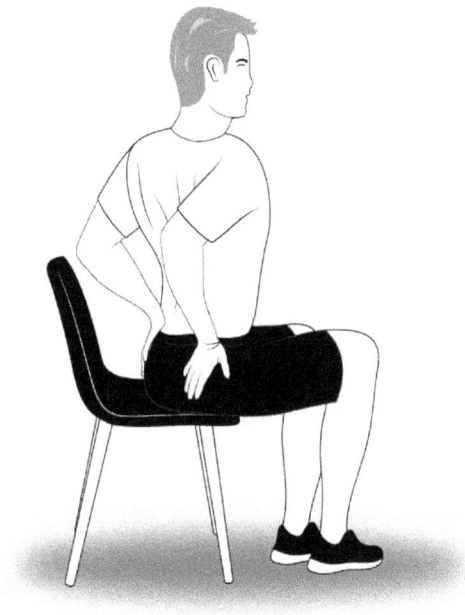

Bicep Curl

How This Helps You

Your bicep is a large, thick muscle located in the upper arm between the shoulder and elbow. Building its strength is essential for a number of reasons such as completing various routine tasks every day, especially those where you bend your elbows. The Bicep Curl exercise is a great way to build this strength so that actions such as carrying the laundry basket and lifting shopping bags are effortlessly performed. Apart from facilitating daily activities and building muscle, bicep curls improve your workout performance and endurance while training your shoulders and overall arm to be more stable.

How to Do It

1. Sit tall in the front portion of your chair with both feet flat on the ground. Alternatively, and just as effectively, this exercise is commonly done while standing.

2. Relax your left arm and let it hang at your side.

3. Place your right forearm on your right thigh with your palm facing up.

4. Make a loose fist with your right hand.

5. Slowly bend your right arm as you bring your fist toward your right shoulder.

6. At the top of this motion, gently squeeze your bicep to ensure a good contraction.

7. Gently lower your arm back down to the starting position.

8. Ensure that the movements to raise and lower your arm are slow and complete.

9. Repeat for a total of 10 times, and remember to contract your bicep each time.

10. Do the same with your left arm.

11. Once you master the exercise, you can add weights to add resistance to your movement. As with any exercise, challenge yourself!

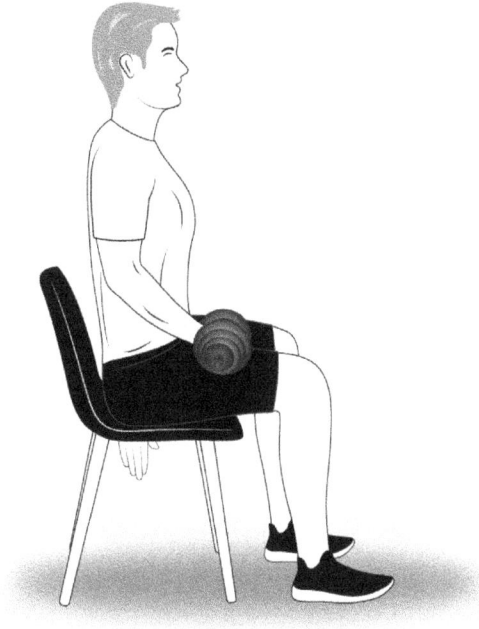

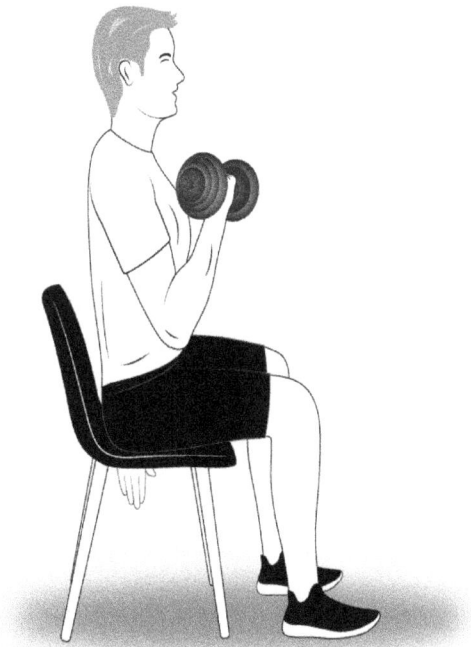

Tricep Push

How This Helps You

Your triceps are the counterpart to your biceps, both being situated opposite of each other in your upper arm. The Tricep Push will help you strengthen and tone these muscles to help you in activities or tasks that require you to straighten or extend your arms or if you have to push anything, such as raising yourself from a chair, closing a door, or pushing a shopping cart. This exercise will directly affect muscle weakness or imbalances in the triceps. Additionally, other muscles enjoying the workout include those in your shoulders, abdomen, and upper back.

How to Do It

1. Sit in a chair with your feet on the ground and your toes pointing forward.

2. Grab the seat of your chair on both sides.

3. Keep your back straight as you gently lean forward very slightly.

4. Simultaneously push down on both arms as if you are trying to lift your buttocks from the chair.

5. Feel and enjoy your triceps contracting as you push down on your arms. Hold the squeeze for a second before you relax by lowering yourself back down onto the seat. If you cannot lift yourself at first, keep practicing until you can do so. Remember that exercise is not a race and that everyone progresses at their own pace. Take it easy on yourself.

6. Repeat the movement a total of 10 times.

7. For an advanced exercise, use a chair with arms and grab onto them instead of the seat. The arms of the chair are more elevated than the seat, which means you have to push harder to lift yourself up.

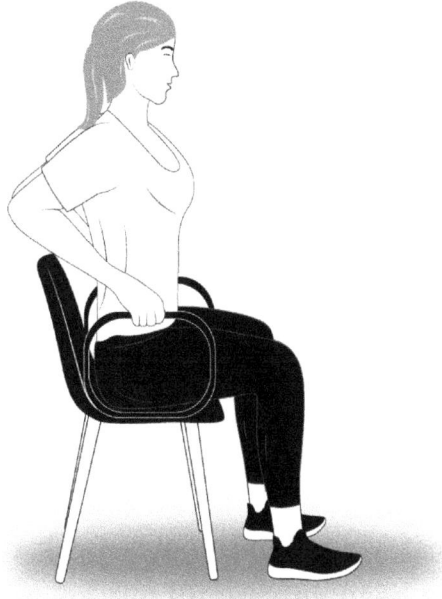

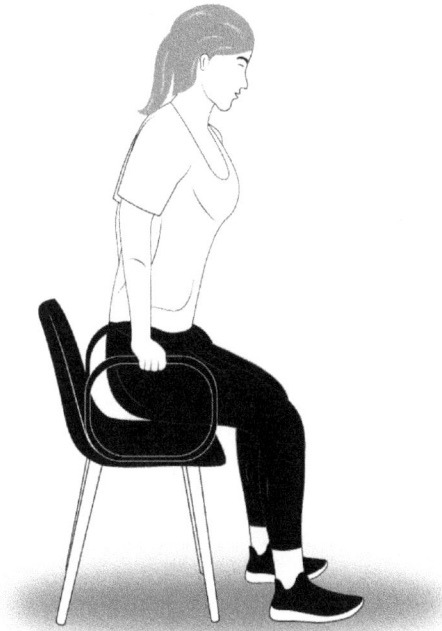

Tricep Extension

How This Helps You

As with the Tricep Push, this Tricep Extension exercise will help you build the arm strength needed for bracing, balance, and fall prevention. In addition, you will find certain movements to be more effortless due to an improvement in your ability to extend and retract your arms. Reaching for cups on a higher shelf, grabbing items from your nightstand, and pulling yourself up from the tub will feel like a walk in the park!

How to Do It

1. Stand or sit tall with your feet shoulder-width apart.

2. Fully extend your right arm upward as if pointing to the sky.

3. Bend at the elbow so that your hand comes back down toward your right upper back/shoulder. As you are bending your elbow, keep your upper arm still. You want your bicep to remain near your ear at all times. Only your forearm should be moving. It may help to do this exercise in front of a mirror to ensure that you maintain good form throughout your movement.

4. Return to pointing straight upwards with your arm fully extended. It is imperative that you still keep in mind your form. You want the transition to be as smooth as possible.

5. Repeat for a total of 10 times.

6. Treat your left tricep to the same 10 repetitions.

7. Once you have mastered the movement and feel comfortable progressing, you can add weights to your moving hand for a greater challenge.

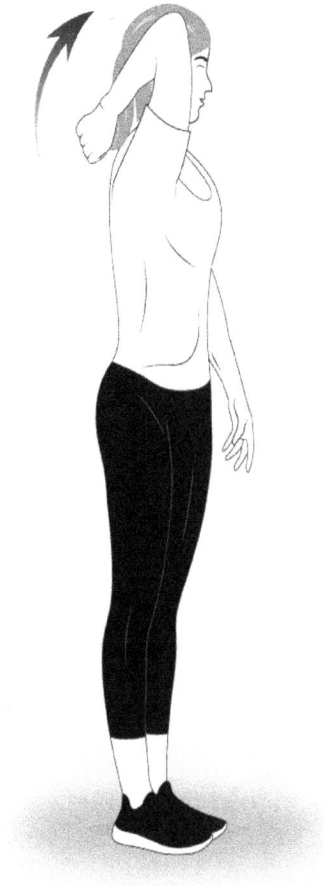

Chest Squeeze

How This Helps You

This exercise, much like Push-ups, will aid in the mobility and flexibility of your chest and shoulder muscles. Although it primarily targets the chest, you will find that your shoulder joints are more stabilized, and your posture is better than ever. Even your breathing will show improvements as an improved posture and more substantial and extended chest muscles support better, deeper breathing. Also, you use your chest muscles for various activities involving lifting, holding, squeezing, and pushing. Therefore, having some added strength will definitely do you good!

How to Do It

1. Stand or sit tall with good posture and look straight ahead.

2. Place your palms against one another, fingers pointing forward, and hold them in front of your chest.

3. Raise both elbows high, pressing your palms together until you can feel your chest muscles contracting.

4. Slowly and in a controlled motion, straighten your arms as you exhale and continue to contract your chest muscles. Hold the squeeze for 2 seconds.

5. Gradually bring your arms back to your chest, still allowing yourself to feel your chest muscles contract.

6. Relax and take a deep breath before repeating the movement for a total of 10 times.

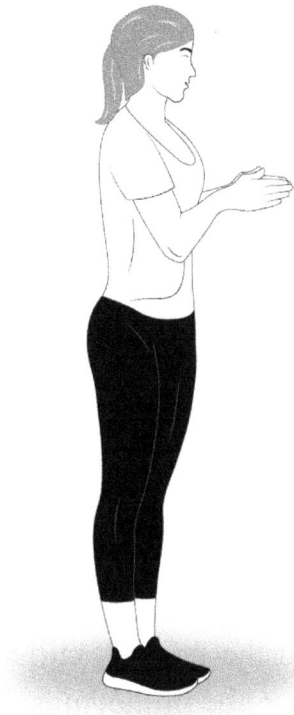

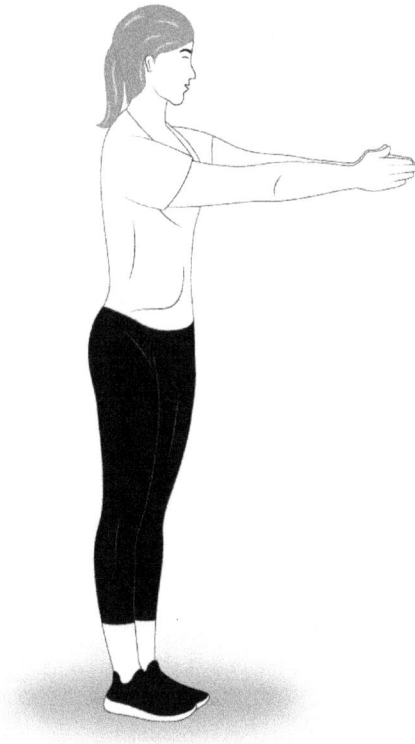

Stomach Crunch

How This Helps You

Working your stomach or abdominal muscles is a terrific way to strengthen your core. The stronger these muscles are, the easier you will find most physical activities, sports, and daily actions, such as leaning over the sink to wash your face. As the muscles surrounding the spine are bolstered and reinforced, your posture, balance, and overall stability will dramatically improve. You will note positive changes such as improved respiratory functioning, reduced back pain, enhanced mobility, and overall ease of daily functioning.

How to Do It

1. Lie comfortably on your back with your feet flat on the ground and your knees bent.

2. Place both hands behind your head to support it as you perform this exercise.

3. While keeping your feet flat on the ground, curl your body up and bring your chest toward your knees. Only use your abdominal muscles to execute the motion, and avoid using your hands to pull yourself up. Your hands and arms should only be used to support your head.

4. At the top of the movement, contract the muscles in your stomach and hold for a second. Exhale as you contract your muscles, and inhale as you relax. If you can only lift yourself a little, that is fine! Keep at it, and you will see improvements over time. Remember that even if progress is slight and slow, it is still progress.

5. Repeat the movement a total of 10 times.

6. If you need to take a break during the exercise, relax at your starting position before continuing. Do the best you can, and I assure you that improvements will soon appear.

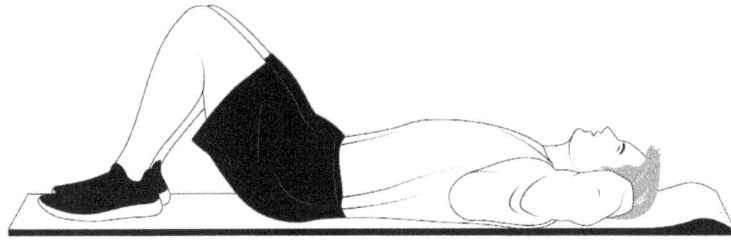

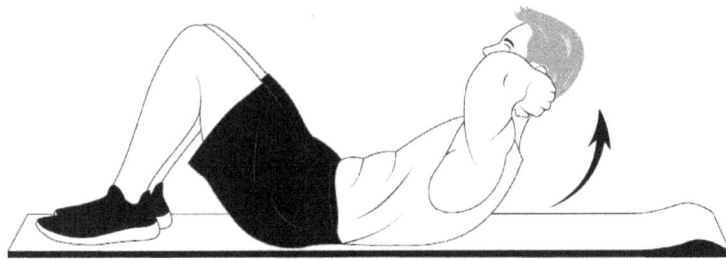

Side Bend

How This Helps You

Side Bends help strengthen the side muscles of your abdominal area, also known as your obliques. Along with the Stomach Crunch, doing Side Bends will enhance your core strength which holds similar benefits as those above. Strong oblique and core muscles are essential for various daily tasks and activities such as getting up from a chair, pushing things around, or carrying items around the home. Your back will be supported, and your overall posture, balance, and stability will be improved. Injuries and falls will be better prevented, while pains and aches will be reduced.

How to Do It

1. Stand tall with your arms relaxed at your sides.

2. Place your right hand on the back of your head, elbow out.

3. Bend at the waist towards your left side as far as you comfortably can.

4. Slowly return to an upright position.

5. Repeat for a total of 10 times.

6. Do the same on the opposite side.

7. You will feel a nice stretch in your side muscles as you lean to the side. The major strengthening of your obliques will occur as you move to return to your starting position. Therefore, do not rush through the motion and try to use only your side muscles to bring yourself back to an upright position.

8. As you advance in the exercise, you can hold a weight in the hand that is at your side.

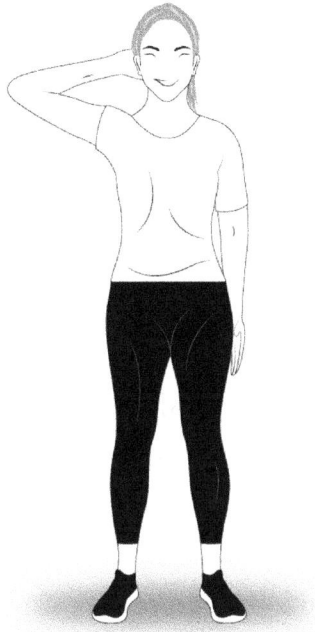

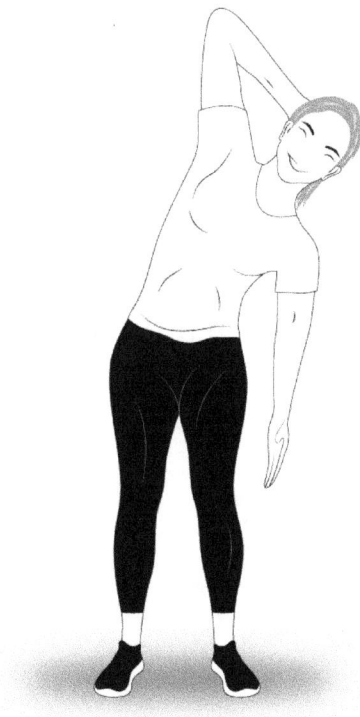

Hand Squeeze

How This Helps You

When you think about it, many daily activities require a good, firm hand grip. In fact, it is the most active part of our upper body (American Senior Communities, 2016). As a result of this exercise, your grip will be strengthened, allowing you to do these everyday tasks such as opening doors, carrying groceries, turning lids, washing dishes, and more. Even peeling an orange requires some strength in your fingers and hands. Also, as you will note, you need your hands for almost all the exercises you do. Therefore, strong hands will lead to enhanced performance and stronger muscles in general. Strong hands are, without a doubt, crucial especially as we continue to age and become more susceptible to conditions such as osteoporosis and arthritis.

How to Do It

1. You can stand or sit, as this exercise is for your hands and forearms only.

2. Spread your fingers on both hands as wide as possible. Feel your hand and finger muscles elongating and the skin on your palms being stretched out. Imagine each finger extending as far as possible and your skin pulling apart.

3. Hold the stretch for 3 seconds.

4. Next, close both hands into fists as tightly as possible. You should feel a good contraction of the muscles, including those in your forearm.

5. Hold the clench for 3 seconds.

6. Relax your hands before repeating a total of 10 times.

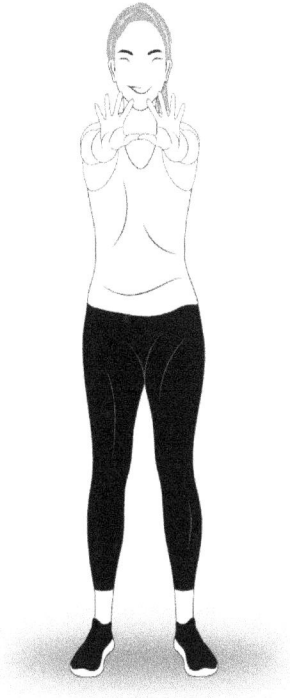

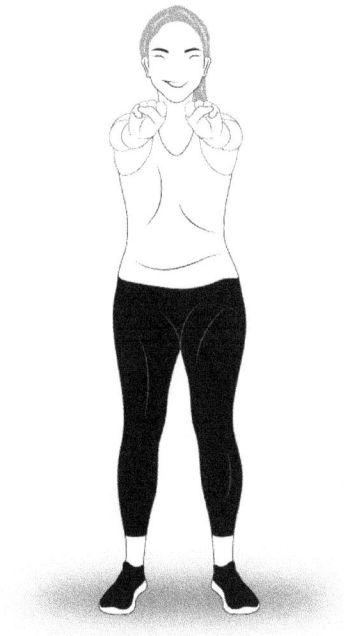

Hand Resistance

How This Helps You

As with the Hand Squeeze exercise above, the Hand Resistance exercise will help improve strength in your hands, fingers, and forearms. You may also see a reduction in pain, such as those associated with arthritis if this exercise is done regularly. By moving and exercising your hands, you will improve circulation and allow fresh, oxygenated blood and nutrients to flow into your hands.

How to Do It

1. For this exercise, you can sit or stand, whichever is more convenient and comfortable.

2. Bring all five fingers of your right hand together. Imagine you are forming the closed beak of a bird.

3. Loosely grasp the front of your "beak" with your left hand.

4. Next, try as hard as possible to open your right hand, using your left hand to resist and prevent your "beak" from opening. You should feel the contraction of the muscles in your fingers and forearm.

5. Hold for 3 seconds before relaxing your hand.

6. Repeat for a total of 10 times before doing the same with your left hand.

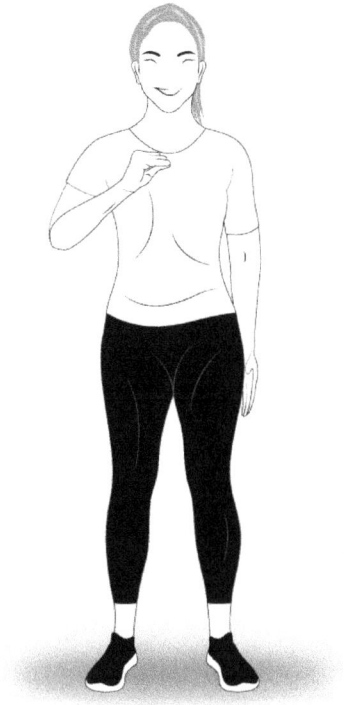

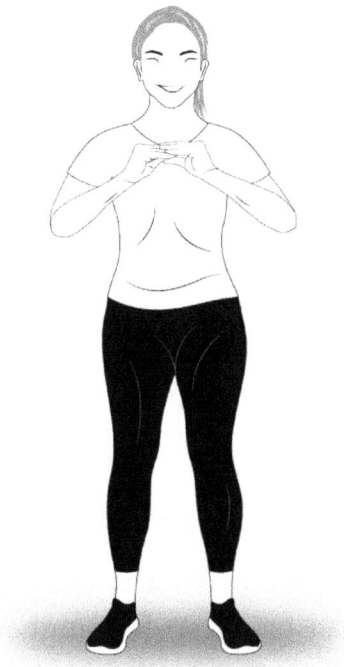

Chapter 8:
Lower Body Strength Exercises

Squat #1

How This Helps You

As we age, our bodies naturally lose some of their strength and elasticity. By doing Squat exercises, you help counteract these changes. This exercise loosens and strengthens supportive tissues, ligaments, stabilizer muscles, and connective tissues. Multiple muscles such as the core, gluteal muscles, thighs, hips, obliques, and calves, are also targeted, and tensed muscles prone to aches are soothed. Blood, nutrients, and oxygen within the body increase while bone density and strength are boosted. This contributes to your overall health by strengthening the lower body and core; building muscle and strength; stabilizing the ankles and knees; preventing pains, injuries, and falls; maintaining balance; and improving joint health, posture, circulation, organ efficiency, flexibility, and mobility. In short, you will find that Squats will help you move and improve for days to come and that routine activities, even just stepping out of the car, will come with ease.

How to Do It

1. Stand behind your chair with both hands on the backrest.

2. Keep your eyes forward, your posture in mind, and your feet shoulder-width apart with your toes pointing forward.

3. Gently engage your core as you slowly bend at the knee, shifting your weight onto your heels, and tug at the hips as if you were going to sit down on a chair.

4. Go only halfway into a sitting position.

5. As you lower yourself, ensure that your knees remain over your ankles, behind your toes, and in line throughout. Also, avoid leaning forward too much, rounding your back, or slouching your head or chest. Remember that good posture is essential in ensuring you engage your muscles properly while avoiding unnecessary strains or injuries.

6. Gently press onto your heels as you straighten your hips and legs back to the starting position. Inhale as you lower yourself, and exhale as you straighten back up. Make sure to squeeze your gluteal muscles at the top.

7. Repeat for a total of 10 times

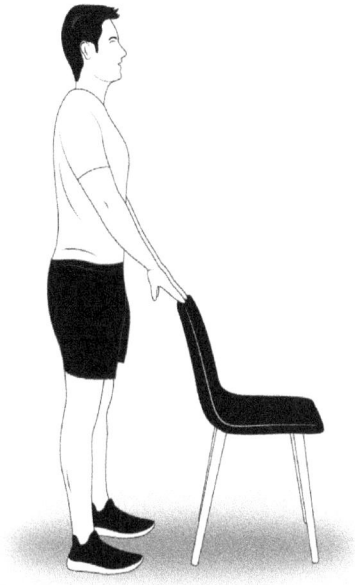

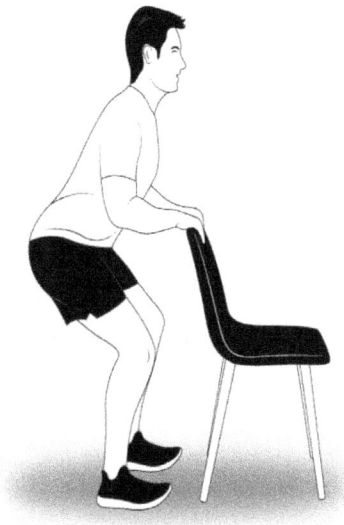

Squat #2

How This Helps You

The following Squat holds the same benefits as those discussed in Squat #1 above, but to a greater degree. The great thing about squats is that they offer endless variations: From different styles and muscle focal points to variations designed to make the exercise easier or harder to match your fitness level, capability, and strength. In this book, all the squats discussed from the first one above to the last below, are considered "basic" squats, so they may initially appear to be quite similar. Their difference, however, lies in their variations of difficulty. Thus, whenever you are ready to do them, the variations within the steps will allow you to challenge yourself and reap the benefits even more.

How to Do It

1. Stand behind your chair with both hands on the backrest.

2. Keep your eyes forward, your posture in mind, and your feet shoulder-width apart with your toes pointing forward.

3. Engage your core as you slowly bend at the knee and shift your weight onto your heels as if you were going to sit down on a chair. Lower yourself far enough so that your thighs are parallel to the ground.

4. Ensure that you go into a sitting position completely this time. The increased difficulty will add stress to your knees, so move slowly and use your hands on the backrest to assist you as needed. Stop immediately if you are experiencing too much pain or discomfort. Keep in mind that you can always go back to Squat #1 and master that movement before coming back to Squat #2.

5. As you lower yourself, ensure that your knees remain over your ankles, behind your toes, and in line throughout. Keep yourself from leaning forward too much, rounding your back, or slouching your head or chest. Remember that good posture is essential in ensuring you engage your muscles properly while avoiding unnecessary strains or injuries.

6. Gently press onto your heels as you straighten your hips and legs to the starting position. Make sure to squeeze your gluteal muscles at the top.

7. Repeat for a total of 10 times.

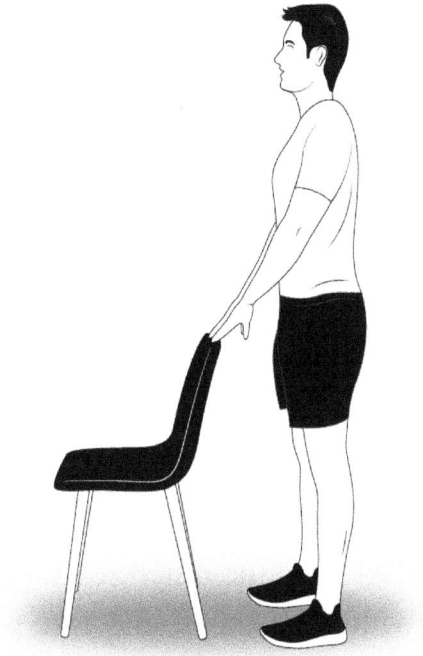

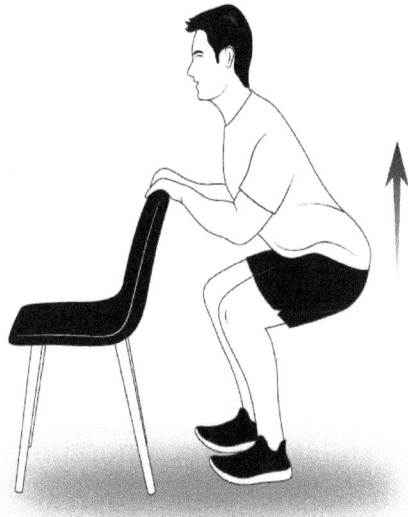

Squat #3

How This Helps You

The benefits of this Squat are very much the same as the first and second Squats above but to a much greater degree. Thus, it affords you more of a challenge and the opportunity to enjoy more benefits.

How to Do It

1. Stand tall with your eyes forward, posture in mind, and your feet shoulder-width apart with your toes pointing forward.

2. Extend your arms straight in front of you, parallel to the ground.

3. This squat does not involve a chair for balance and assistance. Instead, your arms are used to keep your balance. As with the other Squat exercises, be mindful of any pain or discomfort, especially with your knees, and take note whenever you feel yourself losing balance.

4. Gently engage your core as you slowly bend at the knee, shifting your weight onto your heels, and tug at the hips as if you were going to sit down on a chair. Your thighs should be parallel to the ground. If you can only go down halfway, that is fine. You can graduate to the complete "sitting" position as you progress.

5. As you lower yourself, ensure that your knees remain over your ankles, behind your toes, and in line throughout. Avoid leaning forward too much, rounding your back, or slouching your head or chest. Keep your posture in optimal position as you ensure that you engage your muscles properly while avoiding unnecessary strains or injuries.

6. Gently press onto your heels as you straighten your hips and legs to the starting position. Make sure to squeeze your gluteal muscles at the top.

7. Repeat for a total of 10 times.

8. You can practice this exercise throughout the day whenever you need to go from a sitting to a standing position. As much as you can, use only your lower body muscles to get up from a chair or toilet. By incorporating this movement into your daily activities, you will help to bolster your progress in attaining the benefits of this exercise.

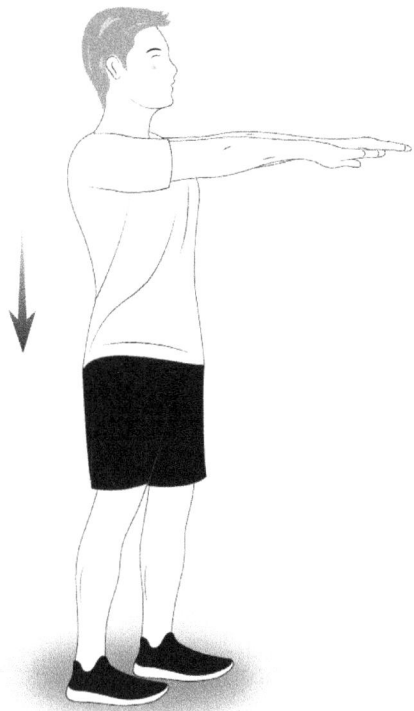

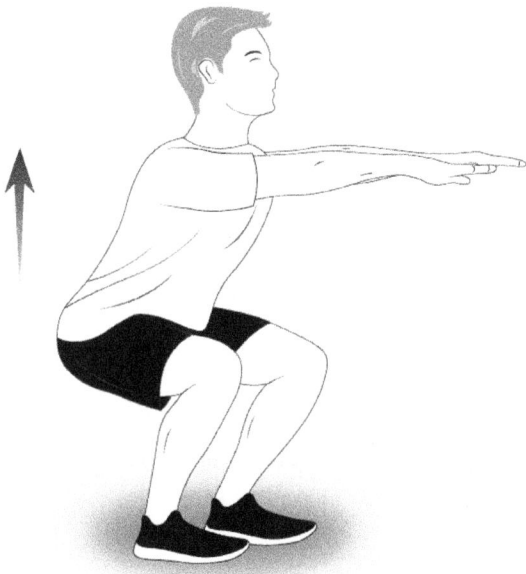

Reverse Lunge

How This Helps You

Reverse Lunges activate several muscle groups, including the gluteal muscles, thighs, and core. They also work on multiple joints by reducing strain and increasing the range of motion. This makes it ideal for those struggling with joint issues such as with the hips and knees. As this exercise improves the health of joints and surrounding muscle tissue, you will find that these lunges improve posture, balance, stability, coordination, flexibility, and mobility. Furthermore, imbalances within the body may be fixed and realigned, injuries may be better prevented, and the chances of falling will be significantly reduced. While Reverse Lunges are not full-body exercises, they are excellent for enhancing your overall frame and general health.

How to Do It

1. Stand behind your chair with both hands on the backrest for balance.

2. Look straight ahead with your toes pointing forward.

3. To ensure that you are targeting your muscles properly, keep your hips squared, posture maintained, and your core engaged throughout.

4. As you are performing the movement, avoid slouching your shoulders, rounding your back, or allowing your knee to pass your toes. This will help you avoid any unnecessary strain on your back and knees.

5. Take a big step back with your right leg.

6. Inhale as you slowly lower your right knee until it almost touches the ground. Feel your muscles as they go through the movements. If you have difficulty going down that far, go only as far as you feel comfortable moving. Progression will occur over time if you keep at it. Keep in mind that this is not yet the difficult part of the exercise. That will happen when you move to return to your starting position.

7. Now comes the actual "working part" of this exercise. Exhale as you make your way up to your standing position. It is very important to keep in mind that the leg doing all the work is NOT the leg that you stepped back with and bent. That is a common misunderstanding with this exercise. The "working leg" is the one in front that is stationary.

8. Repeat for a total of 10 times before doing the same with your left leg.

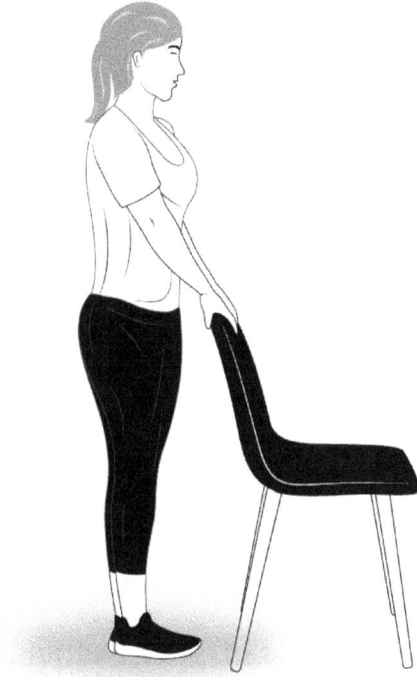
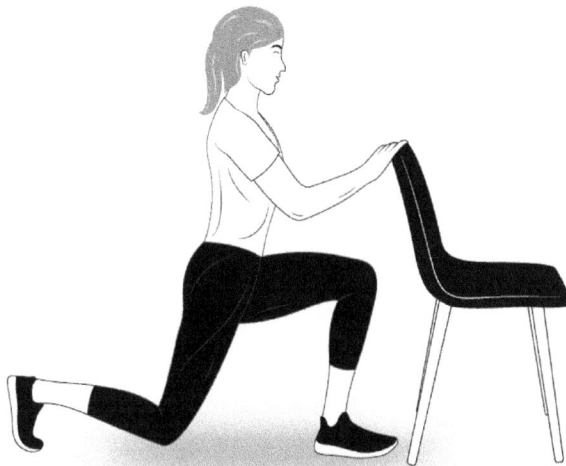

Standing Calf Raise

How This Helps You

By helping to strengthen your lower leg, the Standing Calf Raise will aid in your balance, ankle stability, and overall mobility. Movements that require you to push off with your legs will be easier to do, which aids in acceleration, endurance, and performance. The Standing Calf Raise is also of great aid when it comes to preventing injuries and avoiding falls. You will find that performing explosive movements, such as sprinting and jumping, comes with more ease, which means that you have more freedom to play sports, work around the yard, and dance just because you can!

How to Do It

1. Stand tall behind your chair with your toes pointing forward.

2. Place both of your hands on the backrest for balance.

3. Slowly raise yourself onto the balls of your feet and bring your heels up as high as possible. As you do this, try holding the squeeze in your calves for a couple of seconds. Move slowly and visualize the muscles that are working.

4. Slowly return to your starting position.

5. Repeat for a total of 10 times.

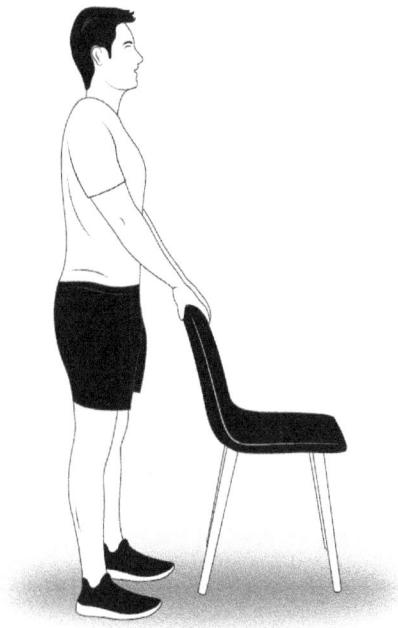

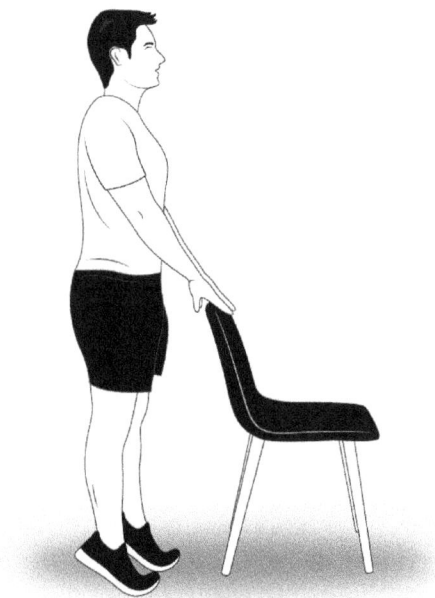

Seated Calf Raise

How This Helps You

The Seated Calf Raise holds the same benefits as its standing variation above. It is also a great exercise to perform while sitting behind a desk, at a table, or even on the couch while watching your favorite show! Furthermore, if the Standing Calf Raise was too difficult for you, this exercise is a great place to start until you can progress to the point of performing it while standing.

How to Do It

1. Sit in your chair with your feet shoulder-width apart.

2. Maintain an upright posture and look straight ahead.

3. Raise both of your heels as high as you can. Do the exercise slowly and deliberately. Avoid "bouncing" your legs up and down while lifting your heels.

4. Hold the squeeze for a couple of seconds, visualizing how the muscles in your legs are working and contracting.

5. Slowly lower your heels down to the starting position.

6. Repeat for a total of 10 times.

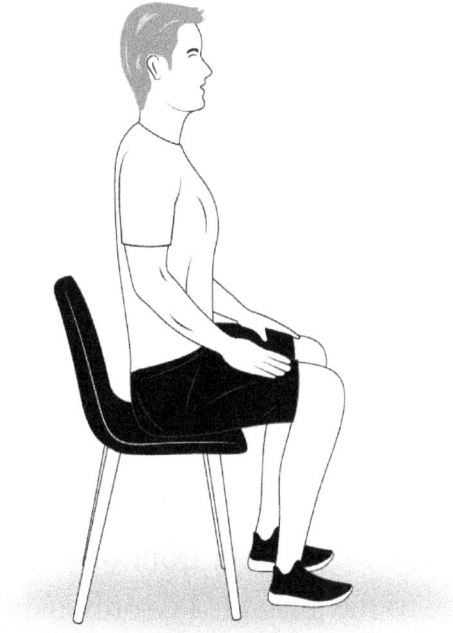

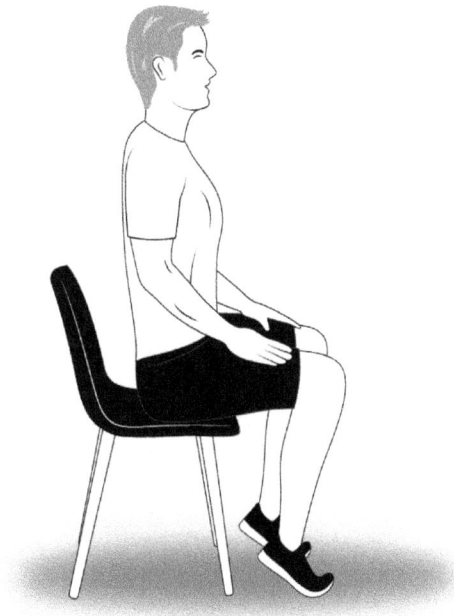

Seated Knee Extension

How This Helps You

Increased strength in the front of your thighs, or quadriceps, will help you retain mobility and independence. It will also help in reducing and avoiding pain in the knees, lower back, and thighs while maintaining bone density, stabilizing the knees, and preventing falls and injuries. Strong quadriceps are also pivotal in enhancing physical performance and supporting you when moving around, sitting, standing, navigating stairs, and lifting heavy items.

How to Do It

1. Sit tall in your chair with your toes pointing forward.

2. Hold onto the sides of your chair for balance.

3. Slowly straighten your right leg out in front of you and lift it up. When you lift your leg, it should be parallel to the ground. Try only using the muscles in your front thigh (quadriceps) to perform the exercise. It is a great way to strengthen your thighs, but remember to do your thigh stretches, too.

4. Hold the squeeze for a couple of seconds before lowering your leg back to the starting position.

5. Repeat for a total of 10 times.

6. Do the same with your left leg.

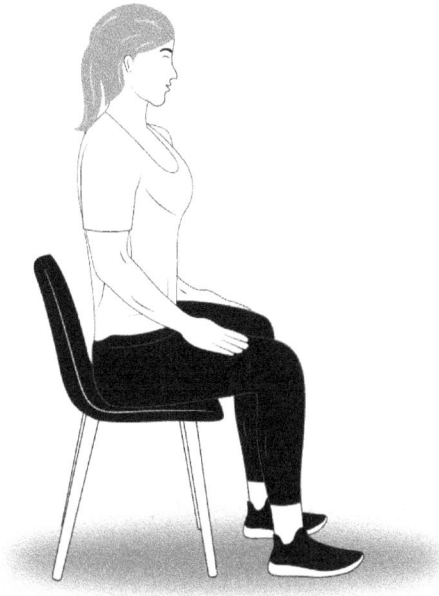

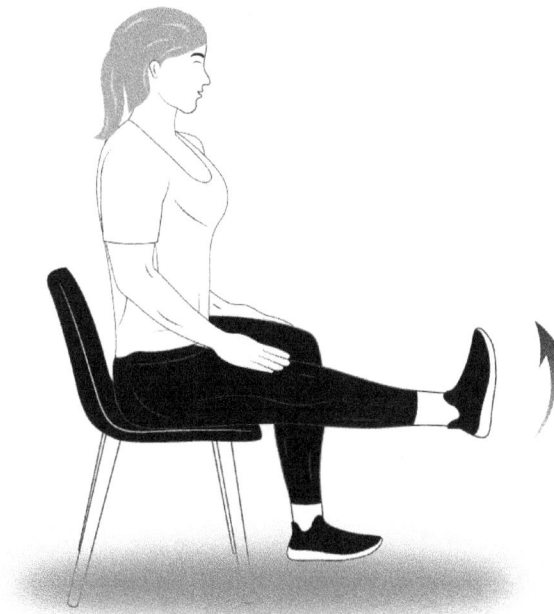

Standing Knee Flexion

How This Helps You

Preventing falls and injuries can be achieved with improved balance and stability by strengthening the back of your thighs or hamstrings. Stronger hamstrings will help you walk with greater ease and will assist in other knee-bending movements such as sitting and picking things up. Along with a decrease in pain, you will notice improvements in posture, flexibility, and overall mobility.

How to Do It

1. Stand behind your chair with both hands on its backrest for balance.

2. With your toes pointing forward, bring both of your feet close together.

3. Keep your left leg straight as you bend your right leg, bringing your heel up as high as you can toward your buttocks. Do the exercise slowly and visualize the muscles in the back of your thigh contracting. Try not to bend your knee so much that it feels like the front of the thigh (quadricep) exercise you have already learned. Instead, once you feel your hamstring being squeezed, know that you are in a perfect position.

4. Hold the contraction for 3 seconds before lowering your leg to the starting position.

5. Repeat for a total of 10 times.

6. Do the same with your left leg.

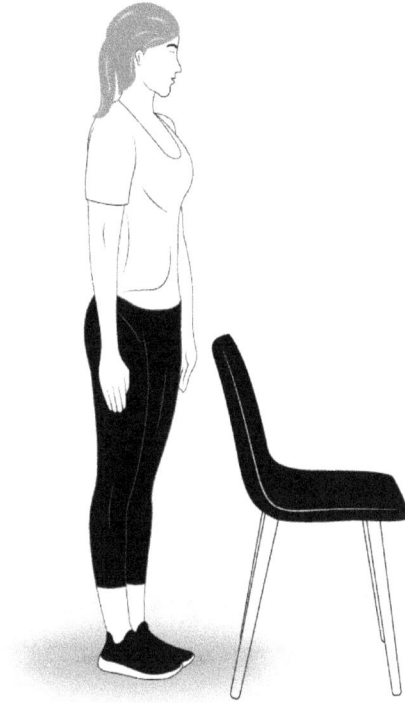

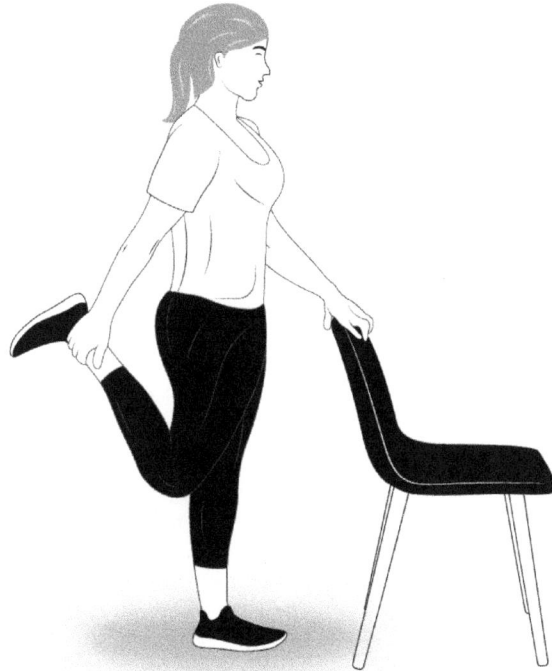

Seated Knee Flexion

How This Helps You

The exercise is a seated alternative to the Knee Flexion exercise above. Therefore, it holds the same benefits to reap, just while you have a seat. Try to think of all the various things you do each day that may involve sitting. Would you be able to do this exercise at the same time? If so, go for it! Ask yourself the same question with all other seated exercises.

How to Do It

1. Sit tall in your chair with both feet flat on the ground.

2. While maintaining an upright posture, slowly bend your right knee and bring your heel as far back and upward as possible. As you perform this motion, ensure that your leg (specifically the hamstring) is the only part of your body moving.

3. Hold the squeeze for 3 seconds. Allow yourself to feel and enjoy the contraction of your muscles. Do not rush.

4. Return to your starting position by slowly lowering your leg.

5. Repeat for a total of 10 times.

6. Do the same with your left leg.

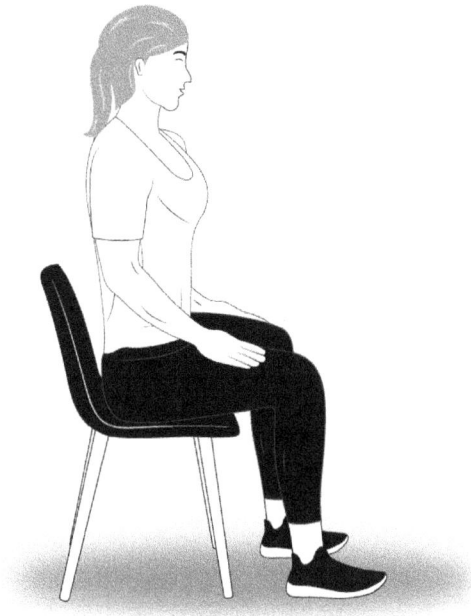
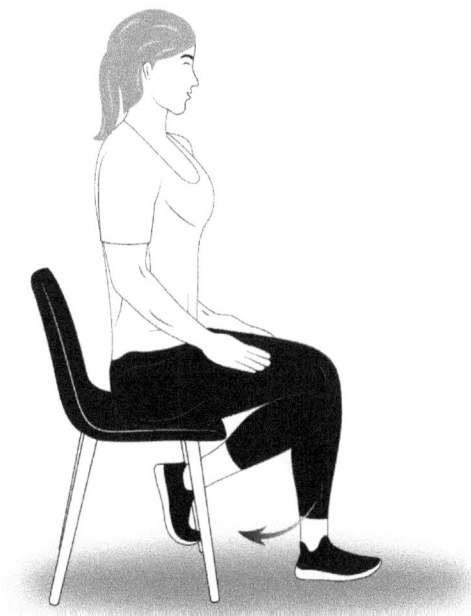

Standing Hip Flexion

How This Helps You

Hip Flexion exercises are great for stretching and strengthening the lower body and reducing the symptoms associated with weak hip flexors and sitting for prolonged periods. Furthermore, the movement will help you manage and reduce pain in the lower back and hips while preventing injuries and falls. You will also note improvements in your posture, core stability, flexibility, balance, and overall athletic performance. Walking, standing, climbing stairs, sitting up in bed, and other daily activities will become more effortless as your body grows stronger.

How to Do It

1. Stand up tall, remembering to use good posture.

2. If needed, feel free to use a chair for balance and assistance.

3. Lift your right leg, bringing your knee up as high as possible.

4. Hold the squeeze for 3 seconds before slowly lowering your leg to the starting position. As you perform the exercise, isolate the movement so that only your hips and quadriceps are involved; feel how they contract and relax as you go through the motion.

5. Repeat for a total of 10 times.

6. Do the same with your left leg.

7. You can also do this exercise lying with your back on the floor.

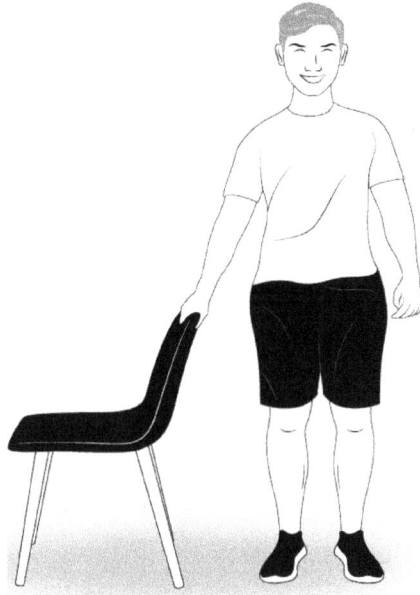

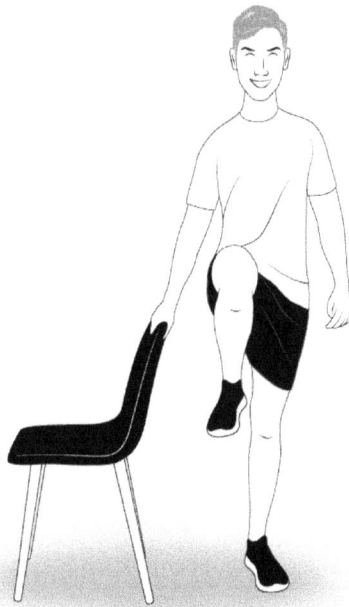

Seated Hip Flexion

How This Helps You

The Seated Hip Flexion holds the same benefits as its standing variation above. This is a good example, as with many of the other exercises in this book, of how even sitting while exercising can help you attain the same great benefits.

How to Do It

1. Sit in your chair with both feet flat on the ground and toes pointing forward.

2. Bend your right knee and lift it as high as possible. While you lift your leg, keep the left leg as stationary as possible.

3. Hold the squeeze for 3 seconds before returning it to the ground. Remember to visualize the muscles you are working on to get the most out of the exercise.

4. Repeat for a total of 10 times.

5. Do the same with your left leg.

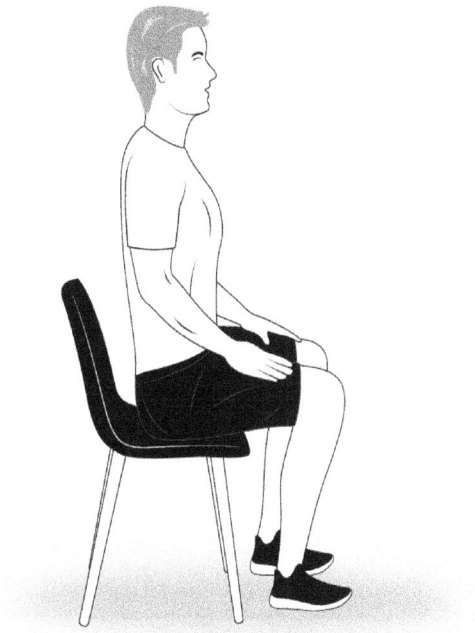

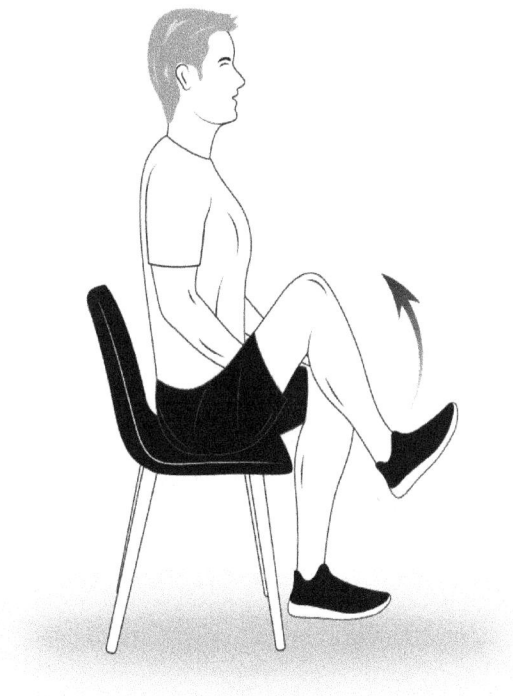

Hip Extension

How This Helps You

Hip Extensions target and strengthen various muscles, such as your buttocks, hamstrings, and hips. When your muscles are more robust, they allow you to remove tension and pressure from your lower back and other surrounding muscles that may cause pain and injuries. Through this exercise, you improve athletic performance, reduce aches, stabilize your pelvis, build core muscles, and give yourself more control over your balance and stability.

How to Do It

1. Stand behind your chair with both hands on the backrest for balance and assistance when needed.

2. Slowly bring your right leg back without bending your knee. As you are doing so, ensure that you maintain an adequate, upright posture and that you are not leaning forward. Your other leg should remain stationary and straight.

3. Feel and enjoy the feeling of your hamstrings and buttocks contracting. Hold for 3 seconds.

4. Return to your starting position by slowly lowering your leg back to the ground.

5. Repeat for a total of 10 times.

6. Do the same exercise with your left leg.

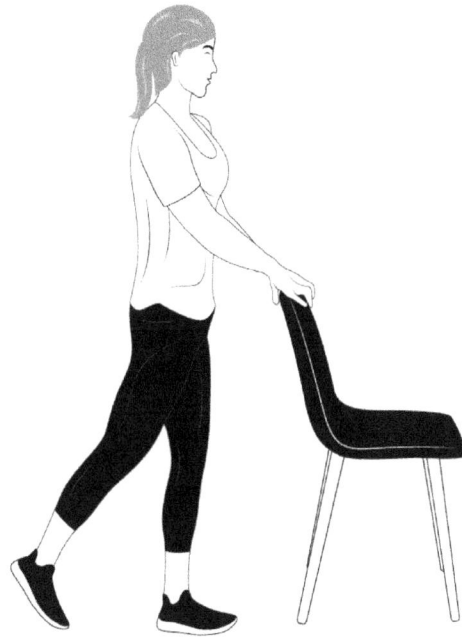

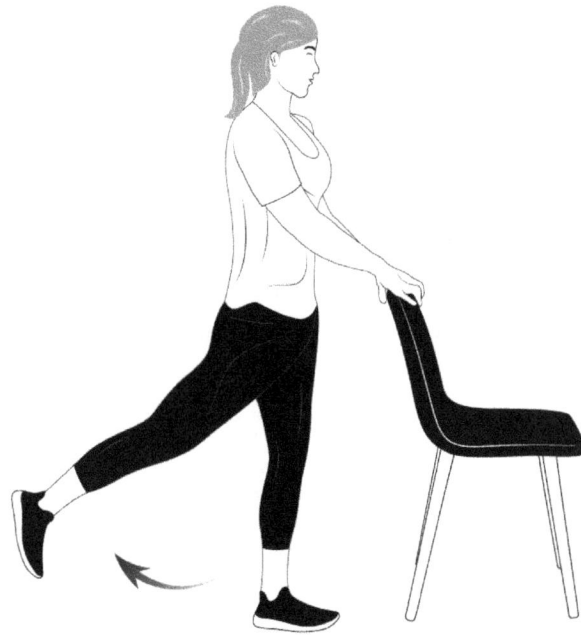

Hip Lateral Raise (Abduction)

How This Helps You

Legs can move away from the body, and joints within the legs can rotate due to our abductor muscles, such as the gluteal muscles. These muscles are essential for keeping us stable and balanced when we walk, stand on one leg, step to the side, and get out of bed. The exercise will allow you to work, tighten, strengthen, and tone these muscles, increasing mobility, range of motion, core strength, physical endurance, and overall ability to walk and move your legs. You will also find that pain within the hips, legs, and knees is significantly reduced and managed. Hip abductors are an often-neglected muscle group. Through this exercise, however, you can rest easy knowing that yours are being cared for.

How to Do It

1. Place your chair by your right side, with the backrest facing you.

2. Place your right hand on the backrest for balance and assistance. Stand upright with both feet pointing forward and look straight ahead.

3. Keep your left leg straight as you raise it outward to the side. Imagine your leg is the hand of a clock, moving from 6 to 8. Be mindful of your posture and avoid leaning on the chair or to either side.

4. Return to your starting position by lowering your leg to the ground or back to 6 o'clock.

5. Repeat for a total of 10 times.

6. Do the same on the opposite side.

7. Performing this exercise regularly will give you the best results. Yet, if you feel uncomfortable with the movement, limit your repetitions to the number you are comfortable with and progress from there. The same goes for all the exercises in this book.

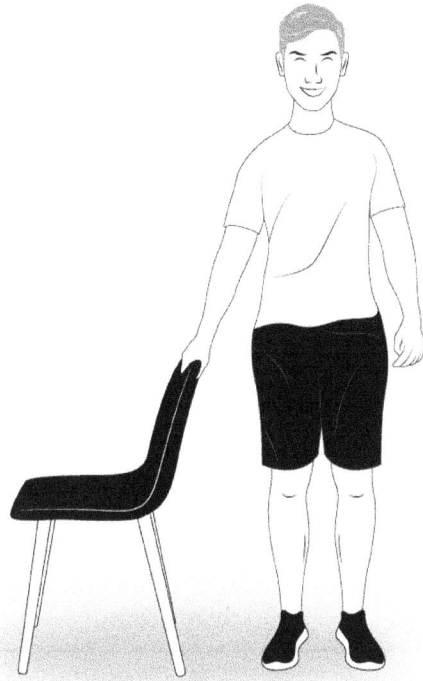

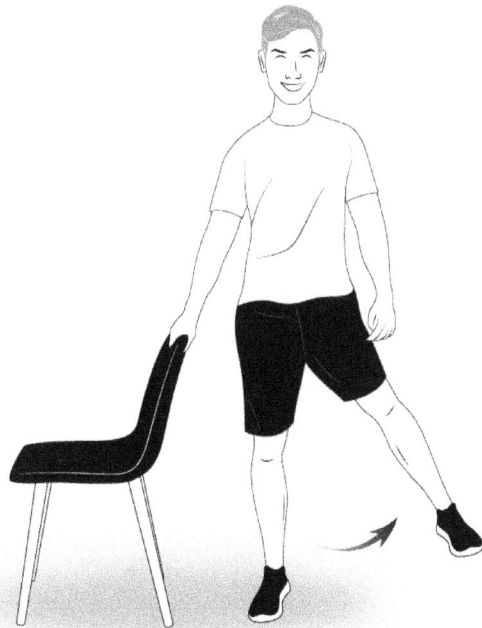

Seated Hip Abduction

How This Helps You

The benefits of the exercise are the same as the standing Hip Lateral Raise above, and as with other seated exercises, it can be done throughout the day while seated anywhere.

How to Do It

1. Sit tall in your chair with both feet flat on the ground and your head facing forward.

2. Place your palms on the outside of your knees.

3. At the same time, try to move both of your knees outward as you press your palms inward.

4. Hold the contraction for 3 seconds while you exhale.

5. Release the contraction as you inhale deeply.

6. Repeat for a total of 10 times.

7. If you have exercise resistance bands, this is a perfect time to pull them out. Simply place them around your knees, where they can act as resistance instead of your palms. Resistance bands come in different degrees of tension. Thus, if you do have them, they can aid greatly in challenging yourself to progress even more.

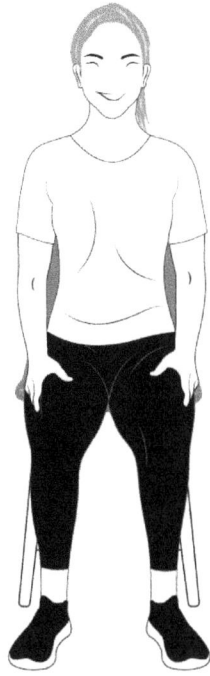

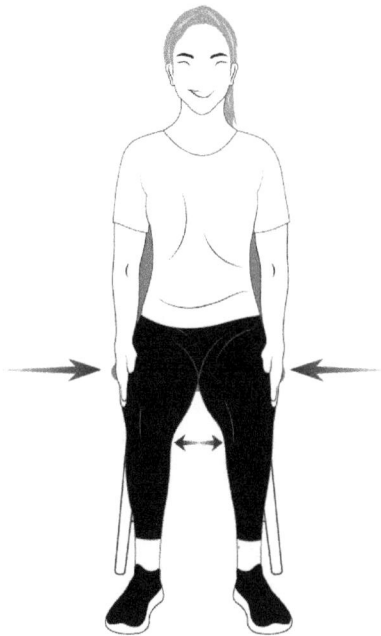

Seated Hip Adduction

How This Helps You

Hip Adductors allow us to bring our legs toward our bodies, in contrast to Hip Abductors, which enable us to move our legs away from our bodies. The adductors are a group of muscles that line the inside of the thighs and help strengthen the hips and lower body. They provide the body with the stability to walk, climb stairs, exercise and do various other activities that we do every day. With age, they help maintain mobility by aligning the hips and knees and supporting the hip joint. As a result, we can avoid falls and injuries while maintaining our performance during physical and overall daily activities. It is clear that by strengthening and working our hip adductors, we can support, care for, and optimize our body's productivity.

How to Do It

1. Sit comfortably in your chair with both feet on the ground and directly under your knees.

2. Between your knees, place padding such as a pillow, rolled-up towel, or bolster. You can use what you want as long as your knees do not hurt during the exercise, and you can get a good contraction on the inside of your thighs.

3. Slowly start pressing inward with both knees, squeezing against the padding. The muscles you feel squeezing are your adductors. Enjoy the feeling of them working.

4. Exhale as you hold this press for 3 seconds.

5. Return to your starting position by relaxing your muscles and inhaling.

6. Repeat for a total of 10 times.

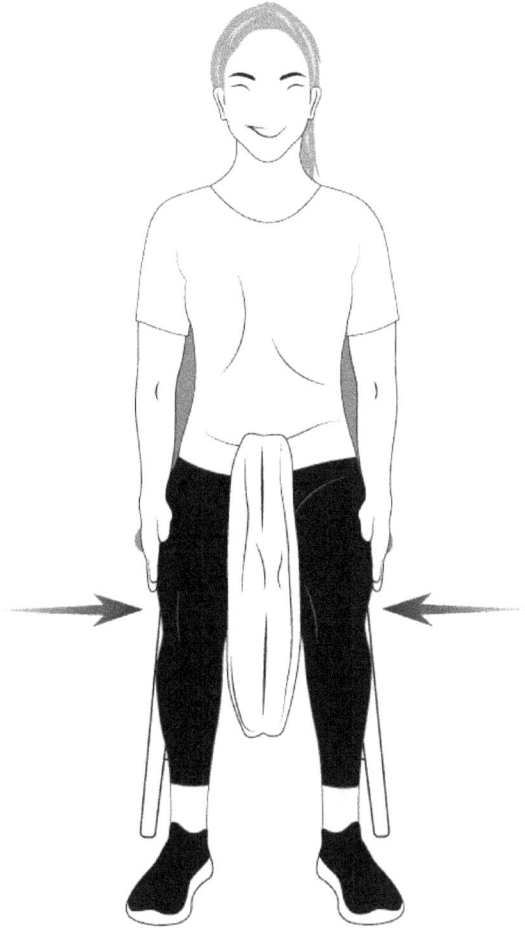

One-Leg Stand

How This Helps You

In everyday life, we go backward, forward, left, and right; sometimes, we even swerve back and forth between directions. All of these movements demand different things from our muscles, not only from our legs. The abdominal muscles, for example, play an integral role in keeping us balanced and stable throughout our walks. Various other activities, such as climbing stairs or standing up from a seated position, require these muscles to be in good shape. This One-Leg Stand exercise is an excellent way to strengthen, tone, and improve the muscles in your legs and core, which will help you improve your balance and stability.

Moreover, how long you stand on one leg can give you an estimate of your muscle strength, balance abilities, and even longevity. People in their sixties can generally balance on one leg for about 20 seconds, while 10 seconds is a great goal for those in their seventies. In summary, the longer you can stand on one leg, the better your muscle strength, balance, and perhaps your longevity are (Araujo et al., 2022). Fortunately, your strength and balance can be improved by doing this regularly.

How to Do It

1. Stand with a chair to your right side to hold onto for balance if needed.
2. Lift your right leg up and see how long you can stand on your left leg. Avoid using the chair unless it is necessary to regain balance.
3. Lower your leg when you can no longer stand on it before repeating with your other side.
4. As you continue to perform the exercise, see if you can increase the time you can balance on one leg and try not to use the chair altogether.
5. For an increased challenge, try closing your eyes while balancing. Many people find it much more difficult to do!
6. If you do this exercise with any partner or group, this would be a fun one to see who can balance the longest.

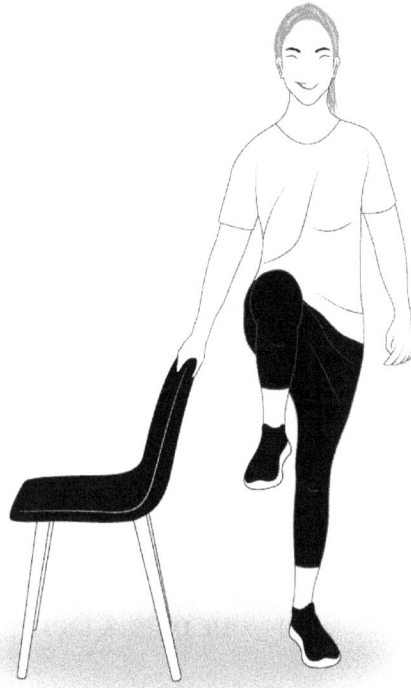
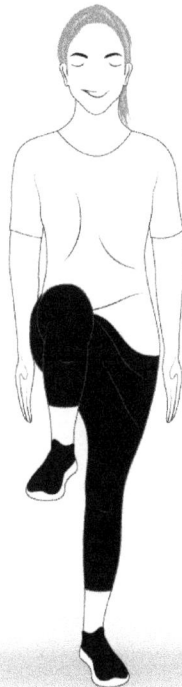

Bridge

How This Helps You

The Bridge exercise is excellent at isolating and strengthening the muscles of your buttocks, hips, and hamstrings. In everyday life, while standing, these muscles help to keep you balanced and stable. Performing the Bridge exercise regularly will help reduce reliance on your lower back muscles when you move and instead rely on your buttocks and hamstrings. Through this exercise, you will experience improved flexibility, balance, posture, performance, mood, and organ functioning with reduced pain in the back and knees. As its name suggests, it will bridge your way toward an improved frame and better capabilities!

How to Do It

1. Lie on your back with your knees bent and your feet flat on the ground.

2. Place your arms at your sides with your palms facing down.

3. Exhale as you lift your hips high, pressing your arms down to the ground. As you are doing so, your knees, hips, and chest should be aligned. Remember to keep both feet flat on the ground during the entire exercise. Avoid "rocking" from side to side.

4. At the top of your movement, squeeze your buttocks tight for 3 seconds before inhaling and slowly lowering yourself down to your starting position.

5. Repeat for a total of 5 times.

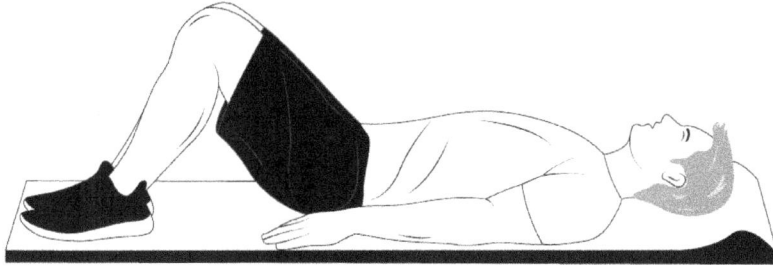

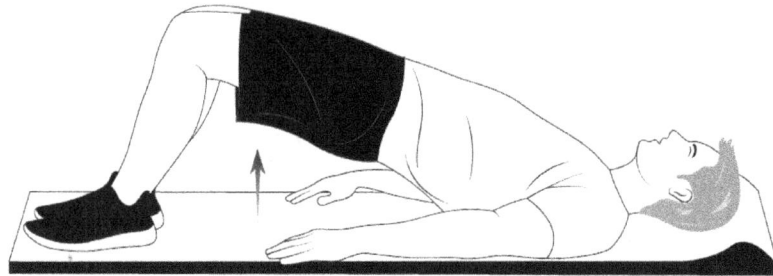

145

Bird Dog

How This Helps You

Although the Bird Dog exercise is challenging, it is excellent for strengthening your buttocks, spine, and abdominal muscles. It will give you greater stability and control over your entire body as it uses your entire frame to target areas such as your core, hips, and back. If you have difficulties moving around or experience frequent pains in your lower back, the Bird Dog exercise will help ease your aches while improving your balance, mobility, range of motion, and posture. This exercise works your entire frame, so it is a great way to remind you of how your various muscle groups come together as one awesome body.

How to Do It

1. Get down on your hands and knees and ensure your back is flat like a table. I would advise using an exercise mat or thick towel for this position, as some floors may feel uncomfortable to your hands and knees.

2. Keep your knees tucked under your hips, your palms down under your shoulders, and your head facing forward.

3. Extend your left leg straight behind you, toes pointing away from your body. At the same time, extend your right arm straight in front of you, fingers pointing forward.

4. When your arm and leg are extended, they should be parallel to the ground and straight. Keep your back straight in your "table" position and avoid slouching or letting it round or fall in. If you find yourself losing balance, lower your leg and arm and regain your stability before continuing.

5. Hold this position for 10 seconds (or as long as you can), then return to your starting position.

6. Do the same with your right leg and left arm.

7. Repeat for a total of 5 times, rotating between your limbs with every repetition.

8. As stated before, this is one of the more challenging exercises. Thus, do not be discouraged if, at the start, you struggle to complete the exercise. As with all the activities, follow the proper technique, move slowly, listen to your body, and build on your progress.

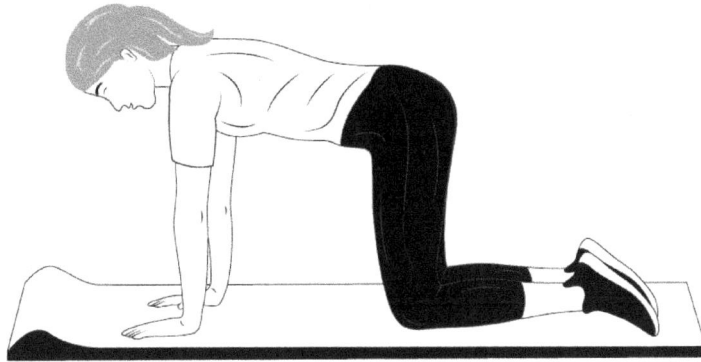
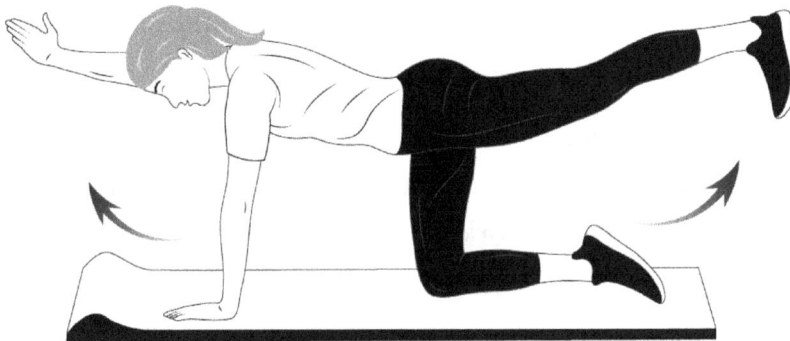

Chapter 9:
3-Day Exercise Plan

With 55 exercises in this book, you may be wondering where to begin, when to perform them, or how to balance them all. Using the following suggested 3-Day Plan; you can start slowly with just a few exercises daily so that your body moves, stretches, and builds strength. Once you start, you will feel confident and comfortable enough to set up your own plan with your choice of exercises and activity combinations.

Beginning with stretching, it may be helpful to consider moving from head to toe, focusing your attention on individual points in your body and loosening them. Afterward, perform the strength exercises (perhaps again following the same head-to-toe suggestion) to develop and strengthen your muscles. You can cool down your body and muscles after the workout by repeating the slow stretches or even going for a nice walk.

When setting up your own exercise combinations, remember to work on all of your muscles throughout the week and to include as many of these exercises as possible throughout your workout plan. Also, when you have worked on one muscle group, such as your shoulders, you may want to rest them for a day or two before working on them again. Resting your muscles is just as important as stretching and strengthening them!

Furthermore, take your time completing these workouts, fully enjoy them, and take in as much as possible as you embark on your own plan and journey toward better health. Remember that these exercises should only be part of your new healthy regimen to eat well, hydrate, take walks, and engage in other physical and mental health activities.

Keep this book close as you work on yourself and your improved life. Remember to work hard regularly and remind yourself continuously that you are not only capable of completing and committing to these exercises but that you are more than worth it, too. As we discussed at the beginning, you live the life you choose. You have chosen this book, and you have chosen to exercise. Those, in themselves, are indicators of progress that have already occurred in your life. Keep going and truly believe that even modest exercise, done consistently and routinely, will give you the great life that you very much deserve.

Day 1

Stretching Exercises

- Neck Forward Flexion
- Neck Rotation
- Shoulder Roll
- Upper Back Rotation
- Chest Stretch
- Hip Flexion
- Calf Stretch

Strength Exercises

- Push-ups
- Standing/Seated Row
- Scapula Squeeze
- Bicep Curl
- Tricep Push
- Squat #1, #2, or #3
- Bridge
- Standing/Sitting Calf Raise
- Seated Hip

Day 2

Stretching Exercises

- Neck Side Flexion
- Shoulder Flexion
- Overhead Stretch

- Upper Back Stretch #1
- Lower Back Extension
- Back Thigh Stretch
- Front Thigh Stretch

Strength Exercises

- Shoulder Press
- Shoulder Forward Raise
- Chest Squeeze
- Stomach Crunch
- Side Bends
- Reverse Lunge
- Hip Abduction
- Seated Hip Adduction
- Standing/Sitting Hip Flexion
- Seated Knee Extension
- One-Leg Stand

Day 3

Stretching Exercises

- Shoulder Stretch
- Upper Back Stretch #2
- Wrist Extension
- Wrist Flexion
- Low Back Side Flexion
- Inner Thigh Stretch

Strength Exercises

- Push-up
- Shoulder Lateral Raise
- Standing/Seated Row
- Tricep Extension
- Hand Squeeze
- Hand Resistance
- Bird Dog
- Squat #1, #2, or #3
- Hip Extension
- Knee Flexion

Conclusion

There you have it! Give yourself a pat on the back for having learned and experienced the stretching, pulling, pushing, and awakening of your magnificent body. From here, with this book still by your side, it is up to you to continue your forward march. Greet each day with optimism knowing that you have stretches to do, strength exercises to sweat through, and, most importantly, plenty of days to enjoy life fully.

You now know what exercise can do for you and how you can reap all of its benefits through stretching and strengthening your muscles. Use your knowledge and do the exercises as regularly as possible; improve with each workout and appreciate every second you spend enhancing yourself and your health.

At the heart of this book are all of the stretches, strength exercises, and benefits set forth in a simple and straightforward fashion. The key to your success is to always enjoy your workouts as you slowly condition yourself toward being more powerful, mobile, and balanced. Embrace exercise as part of your renewed lifestyle and celebrate all that you achieve, even if it is just the ability to bend a little lower or lift a bit higher. Appreciate your journey, your body, and the very fact that you have taken on doing something great for yourself!

As you have learned, there are a number of quick tips on the exercises that will always be there for you to refer back to at any time. Perhaps you have had a bad day and need to refresh your mindset and learn how to embrace exercise once again. Maybe you just need to refresh your understanding of why staying hydrated and breathing properly are important. Or it could be that you have noticed a change in how your body feels and are wondering whether to seek medical attention. Whatever the reason, this book can remain one of the resources in your exercise toolbox to refer to, along with other aids and information you pick up along the way.

This book—*your* book—will always be at your fingertips to consult whenever the need arises. Rather than "Concluding" the book for you, therefore, I will leave it to you to write the remainder of your radiant story. I wish I could be there to help you in person but know that I wish you the best in your efforts and that I applaud you as your biggest cheerleader. My words will always be with you as you work to heal yourself day after day.

Be proud of all the steps you have already taken, of what you will accomplish, and of yourself. You deserve it, after all. If you cannot do some movements or find it harder to exercise on certain days, remember not to be hard on yourself. It might be annoying to hear, but progress does not happen overnight. It surely knows how to take its time, which is why you have to believe in yourself at all times, even when times are rough, and you feel like giving up. *Cliché*, I know, but so very true and applicable.

While this book provides you with all of the basic exercises and information that you need, only you can take the steps needed to run. It is necessary for you to truly understand this. Age does not define or restrict us. We can still achieve anything and everything we put our minds to. Understand and believe this for yourself.

I wish you the very best on your journey, and I know you will do marvelously! Now, go and make travel plans, take more hikes, sign up for dance lessons, and shop till you (almost) drop! Get out there and have a happy, robust life. Remember also that exercise is just one part of your full and active life. Engage in other activities to complement your improved self. Join a gym, treat your body to a healthier diet, take greater care in observing the beauty of nature around you, and spread uplifting vibes to those you interact with.

Now that you have gone through this book, I hope you have found that it has at least nudged you in the right direction toward better health. My goal is to give you the freedom to go forward with fewer aches, more smiles, and better control. I hope I have achieved that.

I will not leave you with a "goodbye" here because I somehow feel that I will always be there with you as you strengthen and flex. I will instead say, as we often do where I live, "Aloha," which is my way of sending you warmth, respect, care, and love. At this juncture in your life, kudos to you for choosing a healthier and happier path.

So how do we answer our earlier question of whether we are at the beginning of the end? The very clear answer is: "No, not even close!"

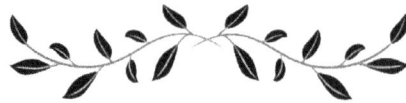

A Humble Request

As I leave you with this book in hand, I humbly ask you a favor as one senior to another. I would be honored and grateful if you would leave a good review for this book on Amazon. Whether you rate with stars or comment on your thoughts and experiences, either would be greatly appreciated. The greater reviews we can get, the better for everyone who needs help. Allow others to improve their way of living and feel the same incredible benefits you get to experience. So, what do you say? Let's help all ripened seniors get up and moving!

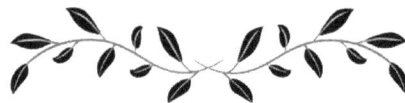

References

Albritton, A. (2020, June 22). *7 Benefits of reverse lunges.* Fitnall. https://www.fitnall.com/fitness/reverse-lunges/

Aletha Inc. (n.d.). *5 Reasons you should strengthen your hip flexors.* Aletha Health. https://www.alethahealth.com/post/five-reasons-to-strengthen-hip-flexors#:~:text=What%20are%20the%20benefits%20of

Alverson, M. (2021, October 10). *Unlock the benefits of neck training: Improve your posture, increase strength, and reduce injury risk.* The Rack APC. https://therackapc.com/reasons-why-you-should-train-the-neck/

American Heart Association editorial staff. (2014). *Balance exercise.* Heart. https://www.heart.org/en/healthy-living/fitness/fitness-basics/balance-exercise

Annigan, J. (2008). *Why is eating healthy important?* Healthy Eating: Sfgate. https://healthyeating.sfgate.com/eating-healthy-important-7166.html

Araujo, C. G., de Souza e Silva, C. G., Laukkanen, J. A., Fiatarone Singh, M., Kunutsor, S., Myers, J., Franca, J. F., & Castro, C. L. (2022). Successful 10-second one-legged stance performance predicts survival in middle-aged and older individuals. *British Journal of Sports Medicine*, bjsports-2021-105360. https://doi.org/10.1136/bjsports-2021-105360

Armando. (2017, August 10). *The (basic) physiology of static stretching.* ACRO Physical Therapy & Fitness. https://www.acropt.com/blog/2017/8/10/the-physiology-of-stretching

Ash, L. (2022, July 26). *3 Key benefits of neck training.* Spirituality & Health. https://www.spiritualityhealth.com/neck-training

Atrophy. (2019, October 7). Biology Online. https://www.biologyonline.com/dictionary/atrophy

Atrophy. (1847). In Merriam-Webster. Encyclopædia Britannica. Retrieved February 02, 2023, from https://www.merriam-webster.com/dictionary/atrophy#:~:text=%3A%20decrease%20in%20size%20or%20wasting,of%20an%20animal%20or%20plant

Atrophy symptoms. (2019). My-Ms.org. https://my-ms.org/symptoms_atrophy.htm

Averill, G. (2021, June 11). *5 Ways to improve your reaction time.* Outside Online. https://www.outsideonline.com/health/training-performance/how-to-improve-reaction-time/

Benefits and importance of back and shoulder stretching. (n.d.). Medi-Dyne Healthcare

Products. https://medi-dyne.com/blogs/posts/why-stretching-your-back-and-shoulders-is-so-important

Benefits of exercise. (2017, August 30). MedlinePlus Medical Encyclopedia. https://medlineplus.gov/benefitsofexercise.html#:~:text=Exercise%20strengthens%20your%20heart%20and

Blumberg, P. O. (2022, March 8). *Build stronger shoulders safely with this subtle shift to lateral raises.* Men's Health. https://www.menshealth.com/fitness/a39369279/lateral-raise-exercise-tip/

Brenner, B., & Eisenberg, E. (1987). The mechanism of muscle contraction. Biochemical, mechanical, and structural approaches to elucidate cross-bridge action in muscle. *Basic Research in Cardiology*, 82 Suppl 2, 3–16. https://doi.org/10.1007/978-3-662-11289-2_1

Bridge exercises: Benefits, how to do it & variations. (2020, April 17). SWEAT. https://www.sweat.com/blogs/fitness/bridge-exercises#:~:text=A%20bridge%20exercise%20isolates%20and

Brisswalter, J., Arcelin, R., Audiffren, M., & Delignières, D. (1997). Influence of physical exercise on simple reaction time: Effect of physical fitness. *Perceptual and Motor Skills*, 85(3 Pt 1), 1019–1027. https://doi.org/10.2466/pms.1997.85.3.1019

Building and maintaining healthy relationships. (2021b, October 27). Healthdirect Australia. https://www.healthdirect.gov.au/building-and-maintaining-healthy-relationships#:~:text=People%20who%20have%20healthy%20relationships

Bones, muscles, and joints (For teens). (2019). KidsHealth Medical Experts. https://kidshealth.org/en/teens/bones-muscles-joints.html

Buzzfeed. (n.d.). *Make perfect Instagram captions* . Pinterest. https://za.pinterest.com/pin/239605642664592198/

Capritto, A. (2020, December 27). *How to do shoulder rolls: Techniques, benefits, variations.* Verywell Fit. https://www.verywellfit.com/how-to-do-shoulder-rolls-for-stretching-techniques-benefits-variations-5087065

Catalyst University. (2019, November 10). *Function of golgi tendon organs [gtos] in movement & exercise* [Video]. YouTube. https://www.youtube.com/watch?v=e5t1EuUG3dE&ab_channel=CatalystUniversity

Cherney, K. (2018, January 12). *Sit-ups vs. crunches.* Healthline. https://www.healthline.com/health/fitness-exercise/sit-ups-vs-crunches#:~:text=Like%20situps%2C%20crunches%20help%20you

Choosing exercise clothes and shoes for seniors. (2022, March 18). Assisting Hands Home

Care. https://www.assistinghands-il-wi.com/blog/choosing-exercise-clothes-and-shoes-for-seniors/

Christmas, C., & Andersen, R. A. (2000). Exercise and older patients: Guidelines for the clinician. *Journal of the American Geriatrics Society*, *48*(3), 318–324. https://doi.org/10.1111/j.1532-5415.2000.tb02654.x

Chrysanthou, A. (n.d.). *The antagonist muscles in a pullup.* Healthy Living. https://healthyliving.azcentral.com/antagonist-muscles-pullup-14164.html

Clare, B. (2021). *The importance of a balanced lifestyle.* Physio West. https://www.physiowest.net.au/balanced-lifestyle/#:~:text=Balanced%20living%20means%20achieving%20optimal

Club, F. A. (2020, May 14). *Can stretching improve body posture?* Fit Athletic - San Diego Best Gym. https://fitathletic.com/stretching-yoga-improve-posture-balance/#:~:text=You%20see%2C%20when%20you%20hunch

Comparative effects of two physical activity programs on measured and perceived physical functioning and other health-related quality of life outcomes in older adults. (2000). The Journals of Gerontology Series A: Biological Sciences and Medical Sciences, 55(2), M74–M83. https://doi.org/10.1093/gerona/55.2.m74

Corbin, M., Vincent, N., & Henderson, L. (2019, March 15). *Ins and outs of weight training.* Penn State Extension. https://extension.psu.edu/ins-and-outs-of-weight-training

Crichton-Stuart, C. (2020, November 26). *The top 10 benefits of eating healthy.* Medicalnewstoday. https://www.medicalnewstoday.com/articles/322268#quick-tips

Cronkleton, E. (2017, October 27). *Thick neck: Exercises, supplements, and more.* Healthline. https://www.healthline.com/health/how-to-get-a-thicker-neck#:~:text=Neck%20exercises%20can%20help%20you

Cronkleton, E. (2019a, September 9). *Neck flexion exercises: Rotation, extension, and lateral bending.* Healthline. https://www.healthline.com/health/neck-flexion#extension-exercises

Cronkleton, E. (2019b, October 18). *Benefits of lunges: 11 Benefits, types, and more.* Healthline. https://www.healthline.com/health/exercise-fitness/lunges-benefits#:~:text=Reverse%20lunges%20activate%20your%20core

Cronkleton, E. (2019c, December 17). *Cooldown exercises: 16 Ways to cool down with instructions.* Healthline. https://www.healthline.com/health/exercise-fitness/cooldown-exercises#for-seniors

Cronkleton, E. (2019d, December 17). *How to stretch tight hips: 12 stretches and instructions.* Healthline. https://www.healthline.com/health/exercise-fitness/how-to-stretch-hips#3-Yoga-Poses-for-Tight-Hips

Cronkleton, E. (2022, February 16). *Bird dog exercise: How to do, variations, and muscles targeted.* Healthline. https://www.healthline.com/health/bird-dog-exercise#alignment-tips

Davidson, K. (2021, August 16). *14 Benefits of strength training, backed by science.* Healthline. https://www.healthline.com/health/fitness/benefits-of-strength-training#benefits

Davidson, K. (2022, March 7). *Battle rope exercises: Benefits and how to get started.* Healthline. https://www.healthline.com/health/fitness/battle-rope-exercises#tips

Department of Health & Human Services. (n.d.-a). *Exercise - the low-down on hydration.* Betterhealth. https://www.betterhealth.vic.gov.au/health/healthyliving/Exercise-the-low-down-on-water-and-drinks#what-hydration-means

Department of Health & Human Services. (n.d.-b). *Heat stress – preventing heatstroke.* Betterhealth. https://www.betterhealth.vic.gov.au/health/healthyliving/heat-stress-preventing-heatstroke

Dolson, L. (2006, March 2). *The role of glycogen in diet and exercise.* Verywell Fit. https://www.verywellfit.com/what-is-glycogen-2242008

Douglas-Gabriel, D. (2016, June 7). *Why grip strength is important even if you're not a "ninja warrior."* The Washington Post. https://www.washingtonpost.com/lifestyle/wellness/why-grip-strength-is-important-even-if-youre-not-a-ninja-warrior/2016/06/07/f88dc6a8-2737-11e6-b989-4e5479715b54_story.html

Duncan, L. R., Hall, C. R., Wilson, P. M., & Rodgers, W. M. (2012). *The use of a mental imagery intervention to enhance integrated regulation for exercise among women commencing an exercise program.* Motivation and Emotion, 36(4), 452–464. https://doi.org/10.1007/s11031-011-9271-4

8 Easy exercises to get a slender neck and shoulder line. (2020, October 3). Bright Side. https://brightside.me/inspiration-health/8-easy-exercises-to-get-a-slender-neck-and-shoulder-line-799134/

8 Foods older adults should avoid eating. (2016, November 29). Sun Health Communities. https://www.sunhealthcommunities.org/helpful-tools/articles/8-foods-older-adults-avoid-eating

8 Upper body stretches to add in your routine. (2021b, September 8). MasterClass. https://www.masterclass.com/articles/upper-body-stretches-explained

Effective benefits of doing upper back stretches for weightlifters. (n.d.). Stretch 22. https://stretch22.com/effective-benefits-of-doing-upper-back-stretches-for-weightlifters/

Effects of overweight and obesity. (2022, March 18). Center for Disease Control and Prevention. https://www.cdc.gov/healthyweight/effects/index.html#:~:text=All%2Dcauses%20of%20death%20(mortality

Eresman, K. (2022). *7 Science-backed benefits of doing push-ups.* Goodrx.com. https://www.goodrx.com/well-being/movement-exercise/benefits-of-push-ups

Esposito, L. (2016, May 26). *MyPlate for older adults adjusts eating guidelines.* U.S. News & World Report. https://health.usnews.com/wellness/articles/2016-05-25/myplate-for-older-adults-adjusts-eating-guidelines

Exercise and immunity. (2022, January 29). MedlinePlus Medical Encyclopedia. https://medlineplus.gov/ency/article/007165.htm#:~:text=Exercise%20causes%20change%20in%20antibodies

Exercise and seniors. (2017, July 26). Familydoctor.org. https://familydoctor.org/exercise-seniors/

Exercise and the heart. (2022). Johns Hopkins Medicine. https://www.hopkinsmedicine.org/health/wellness-and-prevention/exercise-and-the-heart#:~:text=Additional%20benefits%20of%20exercise%3A

Exercise tips for wheelchair users. (2022, October 3). OneStep Digital Physical Therapy. https://www.onestep.co/resources-blog/exercise-tips-for-wheelchair-users#:~:text=Try%20swimming%2C%20rowing%2C%20seated%20boxing

Exercises to help prevent falls. (2022, December). MedlinePlus Medical Encyclopedia. https://medlineplus.gov/ency/patientinstructions/000493.htm#:~:text=Exercising%20can%20help%20prevent%20falls

Fabrocini, B. (2017, November 27). *Posture, mobility and stability - what they are and how to improve.* BackForever - the Movement to End Pain. https://backforever.com/blog/2017/11/27/posture-mobility-stability/#:~:text=Posture%20is%20the%20direct%20link

Ferri, B. (2020, January 3). *Scapula: Anatomy, function, and treatment.* Verywell Health. https://www.verywellhealth.com/scapula-anatomy-4682581

Fetters, K. A., & Bryant, C. X. (2021). *11 Benefits of strength training that have nothing to do with muscle size.* US News & World Report; U.S. News & World Report. https://health.usnews.com/wellness/fitness/articles/benefits-of-strength-training-that-have-nothing-to-do-with-muscle-size

5 Benefits of exercise for seniors and aging adults. (2020, October 25). The GreenFields

Health & Rehabilitation Center.. https://thegreenfields.org/5-benefits-exercise-seniors-aging-adults/#:~:text=In%20the%20aging%20population%2C%20exercise

5 Steps to start a fitness program. (2012, December 16). Mayo Clinic. https://www.mayoclinic.org/healthy-lifestyle/fitness/in-depth/fitness/art-20048269

4 Rowing machine benefits for cardiovascular fitness. (2021, June 17) LifeSpan Fitness. https://www.lifespanfitness.com/blogs/news/4-rowing-machine-benefits-for-cardiovascular-fitness

Freutel, N. (2016a, January 13). *Stretching exercises for seniors: Improve mobility.* Healthline. https://www.healthline.com/health/senior-health/stretching-exercises#:~:text=Seniors%20should%20try%20to%20stretch

Freutel, N. (2016b, August 8). *The benefits and effectiveness of hip abduction exercises.* Healthline; Healthline. https://www.healthline.com/health/fitness-exercise/hip-abduction

Geraghty, M. (2021, August 15). *The importance of personal workout spaces - our gym flooring customer insight.* Sprung Gym Flooring. https://www.gym-flooring.com/blogs/news/the-importance-of-personal-workout-spaces-our-gym-flooring-customers-insight

Gibson, B. (2016, March 1). *Reasons you should do bridges every day.* Fitness 19 Gyms. https://www.fitness19.com/reasons-you-should-do-bridges-every-day/

Gillespie, C. (2020, April 23). T*ight hips: 7 stretches, symptoms, causes, prevention, and more.* Healthline. https://www.healthline.com/health/tight-hips

Good Health Wellbeing. (2017, May 31). *Why breathing properly is so important.* Now to Love. https://www.nowtolove.co.nz/health/body/why-breathing-properly-is-so-important-32690

Griebel, M. (2018, December 10). *5 Benefits of stretching.* Preferred Physical Therapy. https://preferredptkc.com/2018/12/5-benefits-of-stretching/

Hamstrings - strength & flexibility. (2018, December 12). Fleet Feet Sports West Hartford. https://www.fleetfeet.com/s/hartford/sports-medicine/sports-medicine-corner/hamstrings-strength-flexibility

Health benefits of stretching for older adults. (n.d.). LifeSpan Fitness. https://www.lifespanfitness.com/blogs/news/health-benefits-of-stretching-for-older-adults

Healthy Eating Plate. (2019). Harvard T.H. Chan. https://www.hsph.harvard.edu/nutritionsource/healthy-eating-plate/

Hilarious story about the first week working out! (2011). Dustin Maher Fitness.

https://dustinmaherfitness.com/2010/01/hilarious-story-about-the-first-week-working-out/

Holder, J. (2021, July 7). *Calf raise guide: How to do calf raises with perfect form.* MasterClass. https://www.masterclass.com/articles/calf-raise-guide#7KThGOMtBwl9ihvMzQHPgZ

How the lungs work - the lungs. (2022). National Heart, Lung, and Blood Institute. https://www.nhlbi.nih.gov/health/lungs#:~:text=When%20you%20inhale%20(breathe%20in

How to do a shoulder press | Shoulder press variations. (n.d.-a). PureGym. https://www.puregym.com/exercises/arms-and-shoulders/shoulder-press/

How to do front raises | Front raise variations. (n.d.-b). PureGym. https://www.puregym.com/exercises/arms-and-shoulders/front-raises/

How to improve reaction time through physical and mental exercises. (2022, February 2). Biostrap. https://biostrap.com/academy/how-to-improve-reaction-time/

How to set SMART fitness goals. (2022, December 21). SWEAT. https://www.sweat.com/blogs/life/goal-setting

How to stretch your chest: Tips for optimizing chest stretches. (2021a, June 27). MasterClass. https://www.masterclass.com/articles/chest-stretches-guide

Iliades, C. (2018a, January 30). *The benefits of strength and weight training.* EverydayHealth.com. https://www.everydayhealth.com/fitness/add-strength-training-to-your-workout.aspx

Injured man stock vector. Illustration of accident, hospital - 25643758. (n.d.). Dreamstime. https://www.dreamstime.com/royalty-free-stock-photos-injured-man-image25643758

Insomnia - Symptoms and causes. (2016, October 15). Mayo Clinic. https://www.mayoclinic.org/diseases-conditions/insomnia/symptoms-causes/syc-20355167#:~:text=Insomnia%20is%20a%20common%20sleep

Introduction to the Muscular System. (2019). National Cancer Institute. https://training.seer.cancer.gov/anatomy/muscular/

Jackson, P., & Neumann, D. A. (2019). *Sarcomere - an overview.* Www.sciencedirect.com. https://www.sciencedirect.com/topics/neuroscience/sarcomere#:~:text=A%20sarcomere%20is%20the%20basic

Jay. (2010, September 30). *Exercise order - how to arrange exercises in your workout.* A Workout Routine. https://www.aworkoutroutine.com/exercise-order/

Juma, N. (2020, August 7). *155 Self care quotes on the importance of taking care of you.*

Everyday Power. https://everydaypower.com/self-care-quotes/

Kandola, A. (2020, October 1). *5 Glute stretches that may improve mobility.* Medicalnewstoday.https://www.medicalnewstoday.com/articles/glute-stretches#:~:text=Regularly%20stretching%20the%20glutes%20can

Karns, M. (2018, February 5). *How microtears help you to build muscle mass.* UniversityHospitals. https://www.uhhospitals.org/blog/articles/2018/02/microtears-and-mass/

Karthik, K. (2021, December 18). *100 Good attitude quotes that'll boost your self-confidence.* Motivational Lines. https://motivationallines.com/attitude-quotes/

Key, J. (2019, September 18). *16 Benefits of exercise for the elderly.* The Care Workers Charity. https://www.thecareworkerscharity.org.uk/blog/benefits-of-exercise-for-the-elderly/

Khanna, T. (2020, November 12). *How seniors can maintain flexibility through stretching.* The Physio Co. https://www.thephysioco.com.au/the-benefits-of-stretching-for-seniors/

Kutcher, M. (2019, July 1). *Regaining flexibility after 60 - a step by step guide.* MoreLifeHealth. https://morelifehealth.com/articles/regaining-flexibility-guide

Langhammer, B., Bergland, A., & Rydwik, E. (2018). *The importance of physical activity exercise among older people.* BioMed Research International, 2018(1), 1–3. https://doi.org/10.1155/2018/7856823

Laumonier, T., & Menetrey, J. (2016). *Muscle injuries and strategies for improving their repair.* Journal of Experimental Orthopaedics, 3(1). https://doi.org/10.1186/s40634-016-0051-7

Lindberg, S. (2018a). *9 Benefits of stretching: How to start, safety tips, and more.* Healthline. https://www.healthline.com/health/benefits-of-stretching

Lindberg, S. (2018b, June 18). Stretching: *9 Benefits, plus safety tips and how to start.* Healthline. https://www.healthline.com/health/benefits-of-stretching#types

Lindberg, S. (2019, December 17). *7 Best hip flexor exercises.* Verywell Fit. https://www.verywellfit.com/7-best-hip-flexor-exercises-5080772

Lindberg, S. (2022a, March 9). *Does exercise boost the immune system?* Healthline. https://www.healthline.com/nutrition/does-exercise-boost-immune-system#benefits-for-immunity

Lindberg, S. (2022b, August 31). *Benefits of squats, variations, and muscles worked.* Healthline. https://www.healthline.com/health/exercise-fitness/squats-benefits#basic-squat

Live2BHealthy. (n.d.). *Active aging quote.* [Pinterest post]. Pinterest. https://www.pinterest.ph/pin/275212227199877656/

Lower back exercises. (n.d.). Sutter Health. https://www.sutterhealth.org/health/back-spine/lower-back-exercises-stretches

Magalhães, T., Ribeiro, F., Pinheiro, A., & Oliveira, J. (2010). *Warming-up before sporting activity improves knee position sense.* Physical Therapy in Sport, 11(3), 86–90. https://doi.org/10.1016/j.ptsp.2010.06.001

McAlister, L. (2022, August 18). *Staying social as you age.* Encompass Health Connect. https://blog.encompasshealth.com/2022/08/18/staying-social-as-you-age/

McCallum, K. (2020, June 9). *How to Exercise Safely at Home.* Houston Methodist. https://www.houstonmethodist.org/blog/articles/2020/jun/how-to-exercise-safely-at-home/

McCoy, J. (2020, December 24). *11 Benefits of stretching that will make you want to move your body.* SELF. https://www.self.com/story/benefits-of-stretching

Meacham, J. (2022, March 9). *Does exercise boost the immune system?* Healthline. https://www.healthline.com/nutrition/does-exercise-boost-immune-system

Mothes, H., Leukel, C., Seelig, H., & Fuchs, R. (2017). *Do placebo expectations influence perceived exertion during physical exercise?* PLoS ONE, 12(6). https://doi.org/10.1371/journal.pone.0180434

Muscle atrophy: Causes, symptoms & treatment. (2022). Cleveland Clinic. https://my.clevelandclinic.org/health/diseases/22310-muscle-atrophy#management-and-treatment

Musculoskeletal system: Arthritis, lower back pain, bones, muscles. (2022). Cleveland Clinic. https://my.clevelandclinic.org/health/articles/12254-musculoskeletal-system-normal-structure--function#:~:text=Your%20musculoskeletal%20system%20includes%20bones

Musculoskeletal system. (2020, December 11). Cleveland Clinic. https://my.clevelandclinic.org/health/articles/12254-musculoskeletal-system-normal-structure--function

MyPlate food guide (for teens). (2022, April). Nemours KidsHealth. https://kidshealth.org/en/teens/myplate.html#:~:text=MyPlate%20has%20sections%20for%20vegetables

Nast, C. (2021, September 1). *The 30 best workout shoes for every kind of sweat session.* SELF. https://www.self.com/story/best-sneakers-for-all-types-of-workouts#:~:text=When%20it%20comes%20to%20lacing

Nelson, M. E., Rejeski, W. J., Blair, S. N., Duncan, P. W., Judge, J. O., King, A. C., Macera, C. A., & Castaneda-Sceppa, C. (2013). *Physical activity and public health in older adults: Recommendation from the American college of sports medicine and the American Heart Association.* Scholar Commons. https://scholarcommons.sc.edu/sph_epidemiology_biostatistics_facpub/380/

Neuromuscular system. (2021a, June 3). Healthdirect Australia. https://www.healthdirect.gov.au/neuromuscular-system#:~:text=The%20neuromuscular%20system%20includes%20all

Nine easy creative activities to relieve the stress in your life. (2018, November 14). Youthline. https://www.youthline.co.nz/stories/nine-easy-creative-activities-to-relieve-the-stress-in-your-life

9 Hip strengthening exercises for seniors. (2021, January 21). Iora with One Medical. https://ioraprimarycare.com/blog/hip-strengthening-exercises-for-seniors/#

98 Best self-care quotes to remind you what matters. (2022, August 11). Good Good Good. https://www.goodgoodgood.co/articles/self-care-quotes#:~:text=%E2%80%9CSelf%2Dcare%20is%20the%20number

Nunez, K. (2022, January 28). *7 Easy ways to stretch tight glutes.* Healthline. https://www.healthline.com/health/exercise-fitness/how-to-stretch-glutes

Omar, A., Marwaha, K., & Bollu, P. C. (2020). *Physiology, neuromuscular junction.* PubMed; StatPearls Publishing. https://www.ncbi.nlm.nih.gov/books/NBK470413/#:~:text=The%20neuromuscular%20junction%20(NMJ)%20is

Ostrowsky, A. (2019, July 19). *The science behind stretching.* Core Principles. https://www.coreprinciples.com.au/online-personal-trainer2/item/the-science-behind-stretching.html

Parr, B. (2015, March 3). *7 Ways to capture someone's attention.* Harvard Business Review. https://hbr.org/2015/03/7-ways-to-capture-someones-attention#:~:text=To%20get%20the%20attention%20of

Photo gallery: 9 Bad eating habits and how to break them. (2019). Everyday Health. https://www.everydayhealth.com/diet-and-nutrition-pictures/bad-eating-habits-and-how-to-break-them.aspx

Physical activity prevents chronic disease. (2019). Centers for Disease Control and Prevention. https://www.cdc.gov/chronicdisease/resources/infographic/physical-activity.htm

Preiato, D. (2022, January 5). *Build hip strength with adductor exercises.* Healthline. https://www.healthline.com/health/adductor-exercises#exercises

Quinn, E. (2013). *Why a positive attitude is important in sports.* Verywell Fit. https://www.verywellfit.com/attitude-and-sports-performance-3974677#:~:text=A%20positive%20attitude%20can%20help

Quinn, E. (2019). *The basic bridge exercise for core stability.* Verywell Fit. https://www.verywellfit.com/how-to-do-the-bridge-exercise-3120738

Quinn, E. (2022, November 7). *How to do a bridge: Techniques, benefits, variations.* Verywell Fit. https://www.verywellfit.com/how-to-do-the-bridge-exercise-3120738#toc-benefits-of-the-bridge-exercise

Rani, J., Sharma, U. K., & Sharma, D. N. (2018). *Role of adequate water intake in purification of body.* Environment Conservation Journal, 19(1&2), 183–186. https://doi.org/10.36953/ecj.2018.191226

Ravindra, A. (2021, August 10). *4 Unexpected benefits of chest exercises.* Northside. https://www.northside.com/about/news-center/article-details/4-unexpected-benefits-of-chest-exercises#:~:text=In%20addition%20to%20your%20back

Regan, S. (2021, August 27). *This lunge variation works your glutes even more (With less stress on the knees).* Mindbodygreen. https://www.mindbodygreen.com/articles/reverse-lunges

Resistance training – health benefits. (n.d.). BetterHealth. https://www.betterhealth.vic.gov.au/health/HealthyLiving/resistance-training-health-benefits#health-benefits-of-resistance-training

Richter, D. (2020, December 1). *How to train your triceps: Exercises & workout.* StrengthLog. https://www.strengthlog.com/triceps-muscles-exercises-workout/

Robinson, L. (2019). *Senior exercise and fitness tips.* HelpGuide.org. https://www.helpguide.org/articles/healthy-living/exercise-and-fitness-as-you-age.htm

Robinson, L. (2022, December 6). *How to exercise with limited mobility.* HelpGuide.org. https://www.helpguide.org/articles/healthy-living/chair-exercises-and-limited-mobility-fitness.htm

Rodriguez, D. (2009, May 20). *How to lead a well-balanced life.* EverydayHealth. https://www.everydayhealth.com/healthy-living/how-to-live-a-well-balanced-life.aspx#:~:text=Balanced%20living%20means%20considering%20all

Sachdev, P. (2021, June 22). *Health benefits of squats.* WebMD. https://www.webmd.com/fitness-exercise/health-benefits-of-squats

Schultz, R. (2019, June 28). *You've been doing calf raises wrong.* Women's Health. https://www.womenshealthmag.com/fitness/a28209151/calf-raises/

ScienceDirect. (n.d.). *Fascicle - an overview.* Www.sciencedirect.com. https://www.sciencedirect.com/topics/engineering/fascicle

Scott, B. (2021, September 24). *On breathing: The importance of proper breathing when exercising.* YBell Fitness, Inc. https://ybellfitness.com/news/importance-of-proper-breathing-when-exercising#Diaphragmatic-Breathing

Scott, E. (2021, July 29). *17 Highly effective stress relievers.* Verywell Mind; Verywellmind. https://www.verywellmind.com/tips-to-reduce-stress-3145195

Seana. (2016). *Flexibility: Do I really need it?* Freeletics. https://www.freeletics.com/en/blog/posts/flexibility/#gsc.tab=0

Seladi-Schulman, J. (2018, August 27). *Arm: Anatomy of bones, muscles, nerves, and more, diagram, problems.* Healthline. https://www.healthline.com/human-body-maps/arm#bones-and-joints

Shiraz, Z. (2021, July 24). *Build muscle size like tiger shroff with bicep curls, here are its health perks.* Hindustan Times. https://www.hindustantimes.com/lifestyle/health/build-muscle-size-like-tiger-shroff-with-bicep-curls-here-are-its-health-perks-101627101525085.html

Shirreffs, S. M. (2005). *The importance of good hydration for work and exercise performance.* Nutrition Reviews, 63(1), S14–S21. https://doi.org/10.1111/j.1753-4887.2005.tb00149.x

Shoulder rolls | Illustrated exercise guide. (2015, March 12). SPOTEBI. https://www.spotebi.com/exercise-guide/shoulder-rolls/

6 Benefits of abdominal workouts. (2018, October 19). EFM Health Clubs. https://efm.net.au/benefits-of-abdominal-workouts/

Sleep basics: Rem, sleep stages, & more. (2013). Cleveland Clinic. https://my.clevelandclinic.org/health/articles/12148-sleep-basics

Snap Fitness. (2020, October 24). *The importance of hydration during exercise.* Snapfitness. https://www.snapfitness.com/ae/blog/the-importance-of-hydration-during-exercise/

Sports gear: When comfort, fashion and safety go together. (2007, January). Fibre2Fashion. https://www.fibre2fashion.com/industry-article/1235/sports-gear-when-comfort-fashion-and-safety-go-together

Strength training: Get stronger, leaner, healthier. (2021, April 15). Mayo Clinic. https://www.mayoclinic.org/healthy-lifestyle/fitness/in-depth/strength-training/art-20046670#:~:text=Strength%20training%20may%20enhance%20your

Stretching: Focus on flexibility. (2022, February 12). Mayo Clinic. https://www.mayoclinic.org/healthy-lifestyle/fitness/in-depth/stretching/art-20047931

Strudwick, T. W. (2022, January 18). *How to lose weight fast: 9 scientific ways to drop fat.* Medical News Today. https://www.medicalnewstoday.com/articles/322345#science-backed-ways-to-lose-weight

Sweeney, A. (2016, March 30). *Your 6 biggest fitness questions finally get answered.* Redbook. https://www.redbookmag.com/body/health-fitness/a43339/how-to-get-fit/

TedEd, & Dossi, S. (2018, March 31). *What stretching actually does to your body.* TED-Ed. https://ed.ted.com/best_of_web/jRqHvBs9

Tedesco, F. S., Dellavalle, A., Diaz-Manera, J., Messina, G., & Cossu, G. (2010). *Repairing skeletal muscle: Regenerative potential of skeletal muscle stem cells.* Journal of Clinical Investigation, 120(1), 11–19. https://doi.org/10.1172/jci40373

10 Benefits of having an active lifestyle for seniors. (n.d.). Northwest Primary Care. https://www.nwpc.com/5-benefits-active-lifestyle-seniors/

10 Stretches to help your wrists and hands. Healthline. https://www.healthline.com/health/chronic-pain/wrist-and-hand-stretches#:~:text=The%20importance%20of%20stretching%20wrists

The benefits of stretching exercises for seniors. (2016a, January 21). American Senior Communities. https://www.asccare.com/the-benefits-of-stretching-exercises-for-seniors/

Theifels, J. (2017, April 21). *How to breathe while working out, exercising.* AARP. https://www.aarp.org/health/healthy-living/info-2017/breathe-exercise-workout.html#:~:text=We%20need%20regular%20oxygen%20to

The importance of exercise for seniors. (2014, March 23). American Senior Communities. https://www.asccare.com/importance-exercise-seniors/

The life-changing benefits of exercise after 60. (2021, August 30). National Council on Aging. https://ncoa.org/article/the-life-changing-benefits-of-exercise-after-60

The importance of hydration during exercise. (2020, October 30). Australian Fitness Academy. https://www.fitnesseducation.edu.au/blog/health/the-importance-of-hydration-during-exercise/

The importance of proper breathing for your overall health. (2017a, September 26). Elliott

Physical Therapy. https://elliottphysicaltherapy.com/importance-proper-breathing-overall-health/#:~:text=The%20Breath%2FHealth%20Connection

The importance of stretching. (2022, March 14). Harvard Health. https://www.health.harvard.edu/staying-healthy/the-importance-of-stretching

The importance of strong hands. (2016b, April 19). American Senior Communities.https://www.asccare.com/importance-strong-hands/#:~:text=Our%20hands%20are%20the%20most

30 Fun ways to get 30 minutes of physical activity today. (2018, May 6). The State of Queensland (Queensland Health). https://www.health.qld.gov.au/news-events/news/30-ways-to-get-active-exercise-fun

Thurman, M. C. L., Joey. (2022, July 6). *10 Surprising health benefits of squats, from improved posture to better mobility.* Insider. https://www.insider.com/guides/health/fitness/benefits-of-squats

12 Benefits of squats. (2019, April 29). Urban Fitness Solutions. https://www.urbanfitness.com.au/blog/exercise-optimal-health/12-benefits-of-squats

12 Tips to tame stress. (2019). Mayo Clinic. https://www.mayoclinic.org/healthy-lifestyle/stress-management/in-depth/stress-relievers/art-20047257

United States Department Of Agriculture. (n.d.). *Older adults.* MyPlate. Retrieved from https://www.myplate.gov/life-stages/older-adults#nutritiontips

United States Department Of Health and Human Services. (2022, July 21). *Help a loved one get more active: Quick tips.* Health.gov. https://health.gov/myhealthfinder/health-conditions/diabetes/help-loved-one-get-more-active-quick-tips

US Department of Veterans Affairs. (2022, October 27). *Exercise to build healthy lungs.* Myhealth.va. https://www.myhealth.va.gov/mhv-portal-web/ss20181019-build-healthy-lungs#:~:text=When%20you%20exercise%2C%20your%20lungs

Video: Abdominal crunch. (2020, November 20). Mayo Clinic. https://www.mayoclinic.org/healthy-lifestyle/fitness/multimedia/abdominal-crunch/vid-20084664

Villavicencio, A. (2018, August 3). *3 Reasons why staying active benefits the neck.* Spine-Health. https://www.spine-health.com/blog/3-reasons-why-staying-active-benefits-neck

Walker, C. (2015, February 17). *Benefits of backward lunges.* Fitness 19 Gyms. https://www.fitness19.com/benefits-of-backward-lunges/

Wergin, A. (2022, September 29). *Water: Essential for your body.* Mayo Clinic.

https://www.mayoclinichealthsystem.org/hometown-health/speaking-of-health/water-essential-to-your-body#:~:text=It's%20essential%20to%20keeping%20your,hydrated%20can%20do%20for%20you.

What kind of shoes should you wear to the gym. (2022, October). Adidas. https://www.adidas.com/us/blog/612838-what-kind-of-shoes-should-you-wear-to-the-gym

What you need to know about exercise and chronic disease (2018). Mayo Clinic. https://www.mayoclinic.org/healthy-lifestyle/fitness/in-depth/exercise-and-chronic-disease/art-20046049

White, A. (2014, August 22). *4 No-weights trapezius exercises.* Healthline. https://www.healthline.com/health/no-weights-needed-4-trapezius-exercises#bottom-line

Why attitude is important and 11 tips for maintaining a positive attitude. (2021, August 10). Indeed. https://www.indeed.com/career-advice/career-development/why-attitude-is-important#:~:text=Attitude%20is%20important%20because%20it,your%20personal%20and%20professional%20life.

Why is it important to have a regular exercising schedule? (2021, December 3). Buzz Performance. https://buzzperformance.com/blog/why-is-it-important-to-have-a-regular-exercising-schedule/#:~:text=A%20regular%20exercising%20schedule%20lets

Why is it important to have strong obliques? (n.d.). Pilates Fitness. https://pilatesfitness.com.sg/important-strong-obliques/#:~:text=Having%20firm%20obliques%20not%20only

Winderl, A. M. (2022, May 14). *12 Hip stretches your body really needs.* SELF. https://www.self.com/gallery/hip-stretches-your-body-really-needs-slideshow

Yetman, D. (2020a, August 28). *Why does stretching feel good? Benefits and why it feels good.* Healthline. https://www.healthline.com/health/why-does-stretching-feel-good#benefits

Yetman, D. (2020b, September 18). *Full-body stretching routine: How-to, benefits, pictures, more.* Healthline. https://www.healthline.com/health/full-body-stretch

www.ingramcontent.com/pod-product-compliance
Lightning Source LLC
Chambersburg PA
CBHW080801300326

41914CB00055B/1014